W0228046

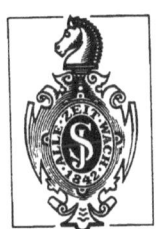

Paul J. Keller

Hormonal Disorders in Gynecology

Translated by T. C. Telger

With 89 Figures and 9 Tables

Springer-Verlag
Berlin Heidelberg New York 1981

Professor Dr. med. Paul J. Keller

Direktor der Endokrinologischen Abteilung,
Department für Frauenheilkunde, Universitätsspital Zürich,
Frauenklinikstraße 10, CH-8091 Zürich

Translator: Terry Telger
3054 Vaughn Avenue, USA – Marina, CA 93933

Title of the original German edition:
Hormonale Störungen in der Gynäkologie, 2nd edition
(Kliniktaschenbücher)
© Springer-Verlag Berlin Heidelberg 1977, 1980

ISBN-13: 978-3-540-10341-7   e-ISBN-13: 978-3-642-81540-9
DOI: 10.1007/978-3-642-81540-9

Library of Congress Cataloging in Publication Data. Keller, Paul Johannes,
1936–. Hormonal disorders in gynecology. Translation of Hormonale Störungen in der Gynäkologie. Bibliography: p. Includes index. 1. Endocrine
gynecology. 2. Generative organs, Female – Diseases. I. Title. [DNLM: 1.
Endocrine diseases – Diagnosis. 2. Endocrine diseases – Therapy. 3. Endocrine glands – Physiology. 4. Genital diseases, Female – Diagnosis. 5. Genital
diseases, Female – Therapy. WP 505 K29h (P)] RG159.K4413 618.1 80-
25866

Typesetting, printing, and binding: G. Appl, Wemding
2121/3130-543210

Preface

During the past 3 years, little has been added to our fundamental knowledge of hormonal disorders in gynecology. Diagnostically, however, there has been an almost complete departure from traditional chemical methods in favor of radioimmunoassay techniques. As a result, diagnostic capabilities which previously were restricted to large centers have now been extended to the office and small clinic. Accordingly, the chapters dealing with these techniques have been revised and updated.

There is also new material on advances in the hormonal treatment of endometriosis and hyperprolactinemic states. Finally, the bibliography has been extensively revised to include a number of recently published books and survey articles of general interest.

Paul J. Keller

Preface to the First German Edition

Menstrual disorders and sterility are among the most common complaints noted by both the specialist and general practitioner. For many patients they are far more distressful than is generally assumed. Recent years have brought great advances in our knowledge. While this has led to major improvements in the results of treatment, it has made it difficult for the nonspecialist to keep abreast of developments in the field of gynecologic endocrinology.

It is hoped that this little book will fill a gap which is perceived by the conscientious physician. Its purpose is not to describe complex pathophysiologic relationships and spectacular techniques, but rather to present a straightforward discussion of the principal hormonal disorders as well as up-to-date methods of their diagnosis and treatment. No attempt has been made to detail the many modifications of these methods, but the selected literature should enable the interested reader to obtain any additional information desired. I am grateful to my close assistants Miss C. Gerber, Miss F. Balmelli, and Miss M. Hubbuch for typing the manuscript and preparing the illustrations, to Dr. W. Koldtiz of Basel for editing the text, and to Mr. K. Münster of Springer-Verlag for his helpful cooperation.

Zürich, February 1977   Paul J. Keller

Contents

A. Physiologic Principles

I. Regulation of Female Sexual Function

The mechanisms governing female sexual function are among the most complex in the human body. It is not surprising, therefore, that they are extremely susceptible to dysfunction. The central regulatory organ is the hypothalamus, which not only contains receptors for all the peripheral hormones, but also serves as a relay point between the endocrine system and environmental influences. It is from here that the "master" endocrine gland, the anterior pituitary, is controlled by the secretion of low-molecular polypeptides called releasing factors. These stimulate the pituitary to secrete adrenocorticotropic, somatotropic, and thyrotropic hormones (ACTH, STH, TSH, respectively), prolactin, as well as the gonadotropic hormones that control ovarian function: follicle-stimulating hormone (FSH) and luteinizing hormone (LH). Follicle maturation, ovulation, corpus luteum formation and, thus, the cyclic production of the principal female sex hormones, estrogens and progesterone, occur under their influence. Estrogens and progesterone are ultimately responsible for the development of the typical female secondary sex characteristics: the growth of the breasts and uterus, the cyclic changes in the endometrium, and menstruation. In addition to their peripheral function, they also exert positive or negative feedback effects on the hypothalamic centers, thus giving rise to a number of closed-loop regulatory mechanisms.

1. Hypothalamus and Releasing Factors

The hypothalamus forms the basal portion of the diencephalon (Fig. 1). It has a low medullary content but is well vascularized. Contained within it are a number of circumscribed nuclei. In the anterior portion are the supraoptic nucleus and the paraventricular nucleus, the probable sites of oxytocin and vasopressin production. The tuber cinereum is situated medially, near the pituitary. The nuclei of this region, which can be collectively regarded as the center of sexual function, communicate neurohumorally with the median eminence and the capillary system of the anterior pituitary via the fibers of the tuberohypophyseal tract (see p 2). Little is known as yet about the lateral nuclear regions.

The regulatory function of the hypothalamus is influenced by numerous afferent connections from the cortex, the limbic system, and the reticular formation of the mesencephalon. Intracerebral transmission is neurohumoral, probably via the

1

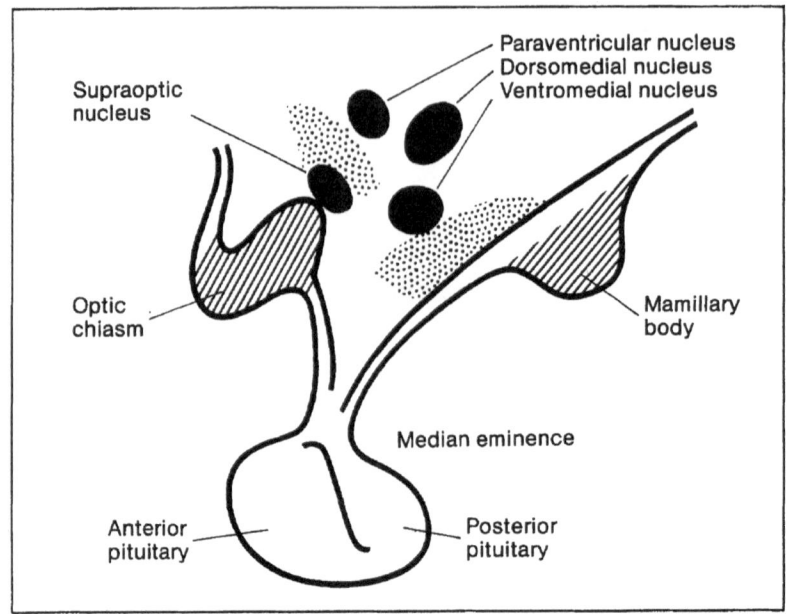

Fig. 1. Hypothalamic nuclei and gonadotropin control centers *(dotted)*

transmitter substances acetylcholine, norepinephrine, serotonin, and dopamine. The hypothalamus also possesses special receptors which are sensitive to peripheral hormone levels (see p 5). Thus, the hypothalamic sex centers are influenced, on the one hand, by continuous sensory input and psychic factors, and on the other, by the function of the ovaries.

The instructions from the hypothalamus to the next subordinate site, the anterior pituitary, are transmitted by low-molecular neurohormones, which have only recently been structurally elucidated and synthesized. The most important of these releasing hormones (RH) in terms of sexual function is that for LH. This factor, termed LH-RH, is a decapeptide with the structural formula

pyro-GLU-HIS-TRP-SER-TYR-GLY-LEU-ARG-PRO-GLY-NH$_2$

and has a molecular weight of 1181. Besides stimulating LH secretion, it also triggers the release of FSH to a smaller degree, thus raising the possibility that LH-RH may be identical with the postulated FSH-RH. The precise nature of these relationships in man has yet to be determined. Inhibiting factors probably exist as well, particularly a neurosecretion which inhibits the release of prolactin (prolactin-inhibiting factor, PIF).

The neurohormones travel through the tuberohypophyseal tract to the median eminence, thereby entering the region of the infundibular capillary network in the pituitary stalk. From there they are transported via the portal vessels of the anterior pituitary to the glandular cells of the anterior lobe, where their main function is to promote or inhibit the release, and perhaps the production, of gonadotropins.

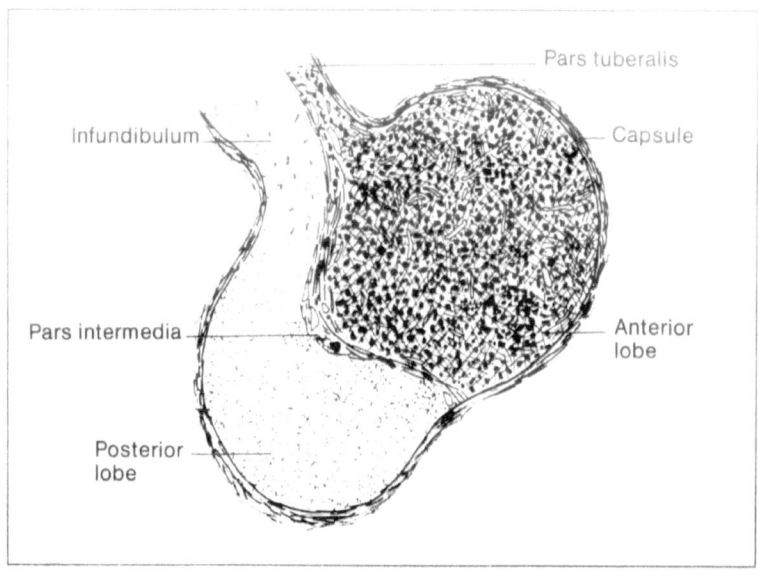

Fig. 2. Schematic representation of the pituitary gland

2. Pituitary Gland and Pituitary Gonadotropins

The pituitary gland, or hypophysis, lies embedded in the sella turcica. It is composed of two main parts: the anterior lobe, or adenohypophysis, and the posterior lobe, or neurohypophysis (Fig. 2), which are separated by an intermediate zone. The pituitary is connected to the tuber cinereum of the hypothalamus (see p 2) by the pituitary stalk.

The pituitary of the adult woman is about $1 \times 1 \times 0.5$ cm in size and has an average weight of 0.5 g. Microscopically, the anterior lobe displays the typical features of the endocrine gland (Fig. 3). It is epithelial in structure, consisting of acidophilic, basophilic, and chromophobic cells, and contains a well-developed sinusoidal capillary network. For a long time it was difficult to associate the various endocrine functions with specific cell types. But now it is believed that human growth hormone (HGH) and prolactin are produced by the acidophils, as evidenced by the development of gigantism in children and acromegaly in adults secondary to eosinophilic adenomas of the anterior lobe. The basophils can be differentiated into subgroups by special staining methods and by the size of their granules. These cells secrete thyrotropic hormone (TSH), the gonadotropins FSH and LH, and probably adrenocorticotropic hormone (ACTH) as well. The chromophobes form an inhomogeneous group consisting partly of reserve elements with no endocrine activity.

The gonadotropic hormones FSH and LH are high-molecular glycoproteins, whose precise structure has not yet been clarified. Their molecular weight is 30,000–40,000. Both hormones contain mannose and sialic acid, and the protein

3

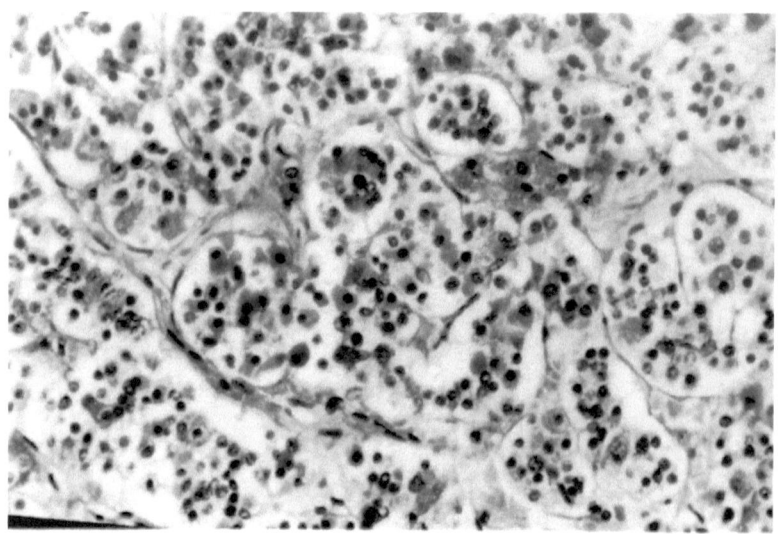

Fig. 3. Anterior lobe of pituitary gland (x 150)

fraction probably consists of 200–300 amino acids. The metabolic behavior of the pituitary gonadotropins is also only partly understood. They are excreted mainly in the urine, the renal clearance differing for FSH and LH with mean values of 0.58 and 0.14 ml/min, respectively.

A third pituitary gonadotropin, luteotropic hormone (LTH), has frequently been postulated, but while it is important in rodents, it apparently plays no significant role in man as an isolated principle. Its identicalness with prolactin, whose primary effect is to stimulate lactation, is controversial.

3. Control Mechanisms

The control of female sexual function is extremely complex. Essentially, it involves a series of self-regulating feedback mechanisms, both positive and negative, which act between the hypothalamus, anterior pituitary, and ovary. In negative feedback, central hormones stimulate the release of specific peripheral hormones, which in turn act to inhibit further central secretion. In positive feedback, central secretions are stimulated by deficient levels of peripheral hormones (Fig. 4). As mentioned, the coordinating center for these as well as central nervous influences is the hypothalamus (see p 2).

Considerable research has been devoted to the feedback loop that exists between the ovarian sex steroids and the diencephalic centers (Fig. 4). Excessive amounts of circulating estrogens (or androgens) and progesterone inhibit secretion of the corresponding RH, thereby suppressing the release of gonadotropins; very low levels of estrogen and progesterone have the opposite effect. One physiologic example of the feedback principle is pregnancy, in which the high placental pro-

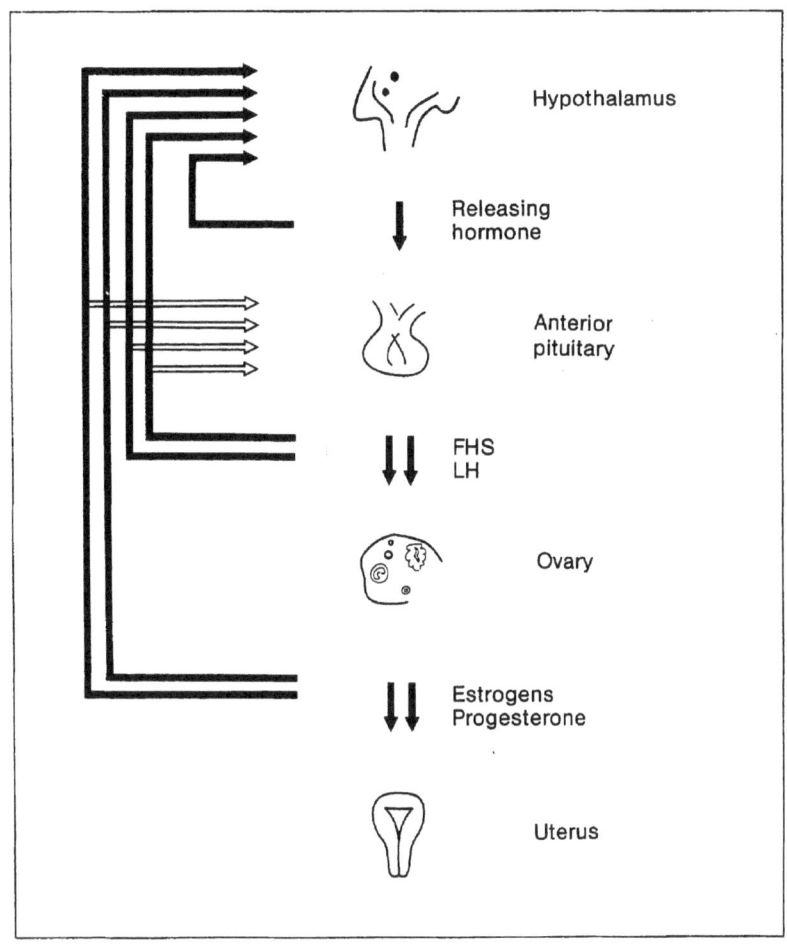

Fig. 4. Feedback mechanisms controlling female sexual function

duction of estrogens causes an almost complete cessation of pituitary gonadotropin secretion. Conversely, gonadotropin production is increased severalfold when estrogen deficiency develops secondary to the loss of ovarian function (see p 18). This feedback mechanism is exploited clinically by the use of synthetic estrogens and gestagens to suppress the midcycle LH peak and thus inhibit ovulation. On the other hand, the administration of low doses of certain sex steroids can stimulate gonadotropin secretion, thus providing a means of inducing ovulation. There are probably a number of other feedback loops. For example, the gonadotropins themselves probably act on the hypothalamic centers by a "short feedback" mechanism. Perhaps the RH even regulate their own secretion through an "ultrashort" loop (Fig. 4).

II. The Menstrual Cycle

1. Ovary and Ovum

The ovary is a paired organ, each of which measure about $3 \times 2 \times 1$ cm in women of reproductive age. The average weight of the ovary is 7–14 g. All but the hilus is located within the peritoneal cavity. Each ovary is joined to the uterus by the ovarian ligament and receives its vascular supply through the infundibulopelvic ligament. The ovary is enclosed by the tough tunica albuginea, below which is the actual germinal parenchyma with the follicles. The interior of the ovary consists of a medullary zone containing mainly nerves and blood vessels (Fig. 5).

The primordial germ cells in the germinal epithelium of the ovary, called the oogonia, migrate from the allantois into the germinal tract at about the 8th week of gestation. Between the 10th and 20th weeks of gestation, they differentiate into oocytes and simultaneously undergo rapid mitotic division. These oocytes then become surrounded by a single layer of cubic cells, called the follicle cells, thereby forming the primordial follicles. Initially there are several million of these follicles, each about 0.05 mm in diameter. But progressive atresia in fetal life reduces their number, leaving about 500,000–700,000 in the newborn female. In some cases primary follicles (Fig. 6) have already started to form during childhood through enlargement of the oocytes. Atresia continues, meanwhile, and by puberty the number of follicles is reduced by approximately half.

With the onset of puberty the follicle cells grow and multiply under the influence of increasing gonadotropin secretion, and a multilayered membrana granulosa develops. The oocyte itself also enlarges to a full 0.1 mm in diameter, becoming the largest cell in the body, and is now called a secondary follicle (Fig. 7). The

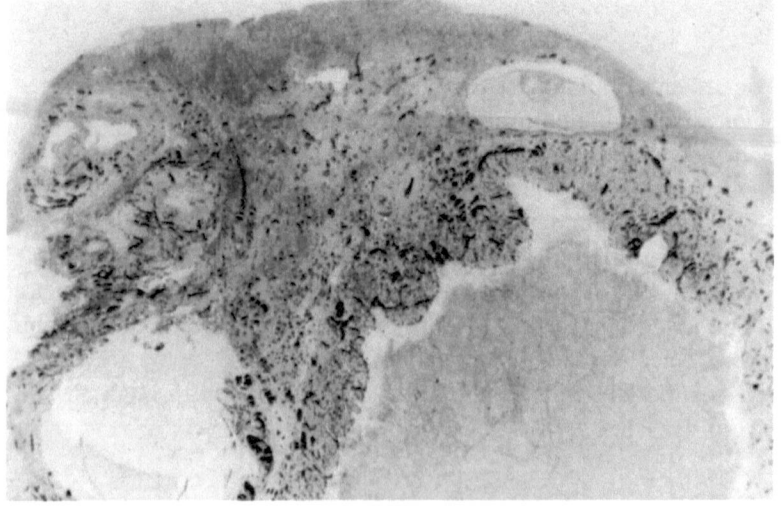

Fig. 5. Section of ovary in normal mature woman (x 1.5)

secondary follicle develops into a tertiary or vesicular follicle, characterized by the presence of a fluid-filled cavity (Fig. 8). The membrana granulosa, which now has many layers, thickens at one point and protrudes into the follicular cavity as the cumulus oopherus, which surrounds the ovum. The connective tissue adjacent to the follicle differentiates into the extensively vascularized internal and external tunica.

Finally, individual tertiary follicles develop into mature Graafian follicles, which can reach more than 2 cm in diameter. Shortly before ovulation the ovum under-

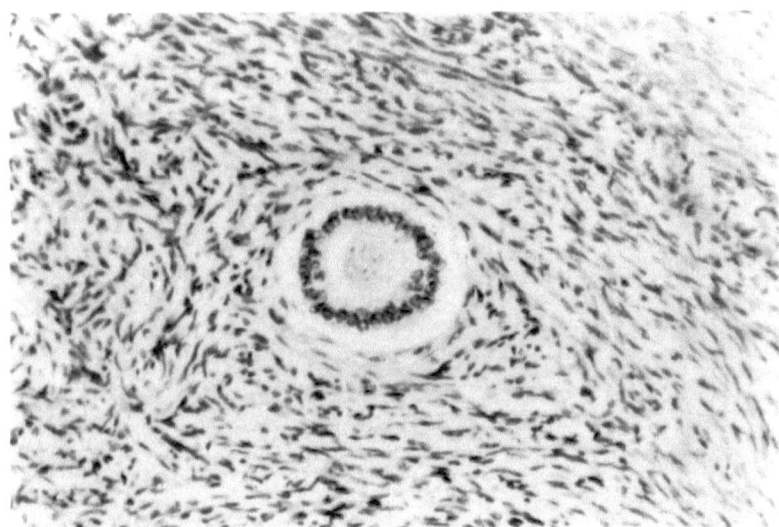

Fig. 6. Primary follicle (x 60)

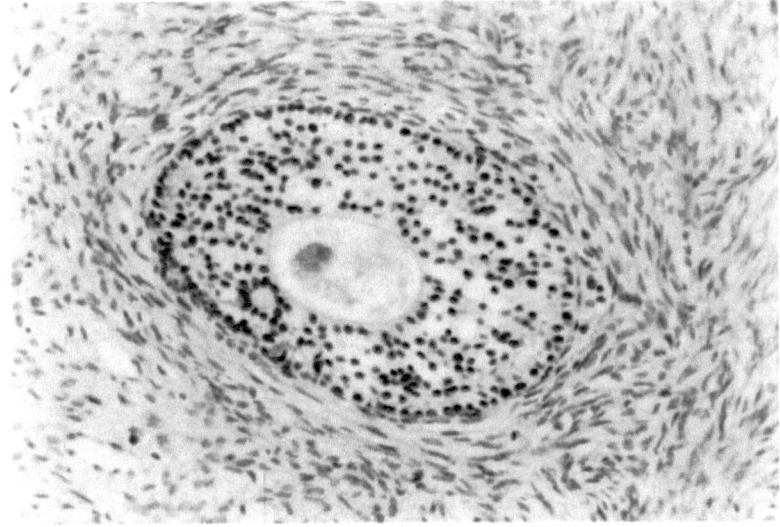

Fig. 7. Secondary follicle (x 60)

goes its first meiosis. The pressure within the follicle builds rapidly while proteolytic enzymes in the follicular fluid attack the follicle wall. Finally the wall ruptures, causing expulsion of the ovum together with its surrounding cells and follicular fluid. Aided by the fimbrial current and tubal peristalsis, the ovum travels through the infundibulum into the ampulla of the Fallopian tube; the second meiosis takes place at this point. Under favorable conditions, fertilization occurs (see p 14). Otherwise the ovum still enters the uterus, but is expelled about 2 weeks later with the menstrual flow.

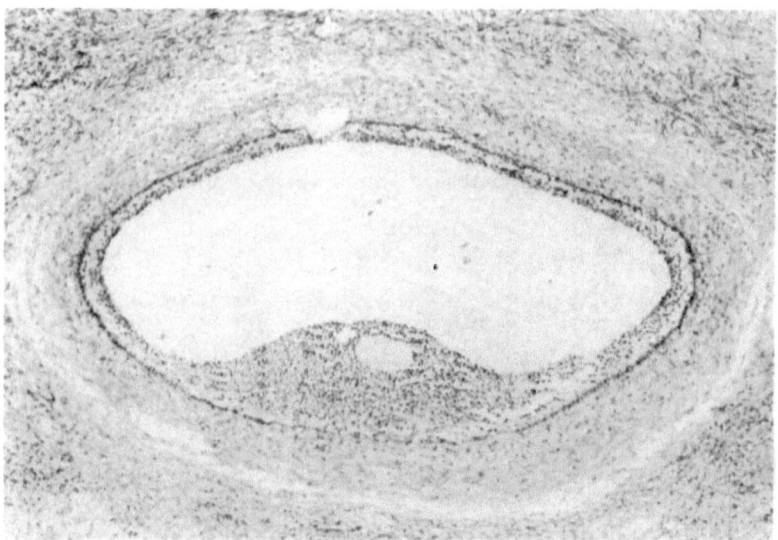

Fig. 8. Tertiary follicle (x 15)

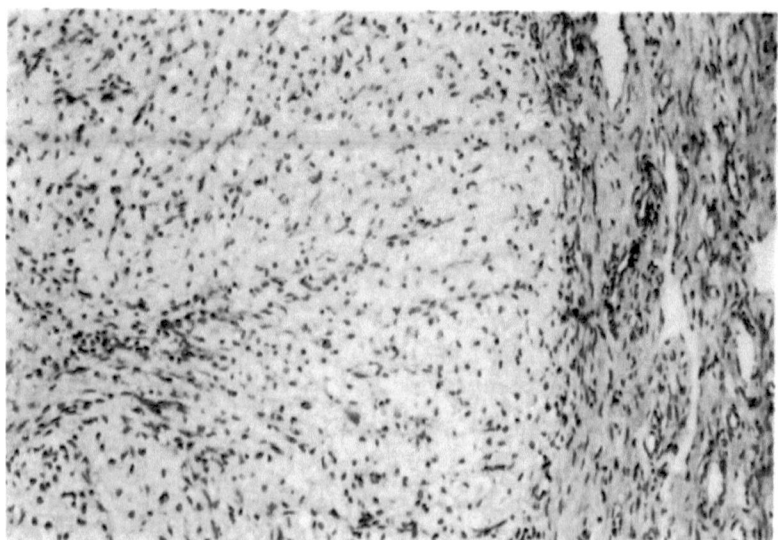

Fig. 9. Corpus luteum (x 15)

Immediately after ovulation the granulosa and theca cells of the ruptured follicle again start to proliferate under the influence of LH. Lipids become concentrated in these cells, and a rich vascularity develops. The resulting structure, called the corpus luteum (Fig. 9), reaches its "full bloom" in 3–7 days. After about 10 days, unless impregnation has occurred, the corpus luteum rapidly regresses by a process of hyaline degeneration; after about 2 months all that remains is a fibrous tissue scar, the corpus albicans.

Since ovulation recurs every 4 weeks on the average, only about 400 primordial follicles reach maturity during the reproductive years; the rest become atretic. A few thousand primordial follicles are still present at menopause, but they have become largely unresponsive to the gonadotropins.

2. Female Sex Hormones

a) Chemistry and Biosynthesis

The granulosa cells and theca cells produce a number of sex hormones, the most important of which are estrone, estradiol, estriol, progesterone, 17α-hydroxy-progesterone, dehydroepiandrosterone, and androstenedione, as well as testosterone. Chemically, the three estrogens are C_{18} steroids, the gestagens progesterone and 17α-hydroxyprogesterone are C_{21} steroids, and the androgens are C_{19} steroids. In each case the corresponding number of carbon atoms are bound in a framework of three hydrated benzene rings and a cyclopentanophenanthrene ring (Figs. 10–13).

The biosynthesis of these hormones takes place under the influence of the pituitary gonadotropins FSH and LH. The starting material is always activated acetate, three molecules of which combine to form mevalonic acid. From this is formed squalene, a C_{30} compound which is transformed first into lanosterol, then into cholesterol. Following oxidative cleavage of isocaproic acid and three CO_2 groups, the biologically inactive product pregnenolone is formed. Dehydration then yields progesterone, which is formed principally by the corpus luteum and which plays a pivotal role in steroid metabolism. From here the pathway leads to 17α-hydroxy-progesterone, and then to androstenedione (Fig. 14), which in turn gives rise to testosterone on the one hand, or to estrone, estradiol, and estriol on the other.

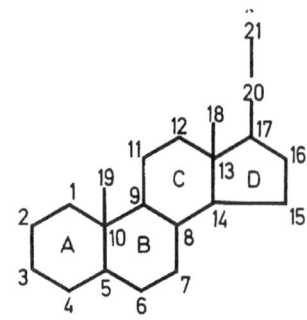

Fig. 10. Basic structure of steroid hormones; rings and carbon atoms are labeled

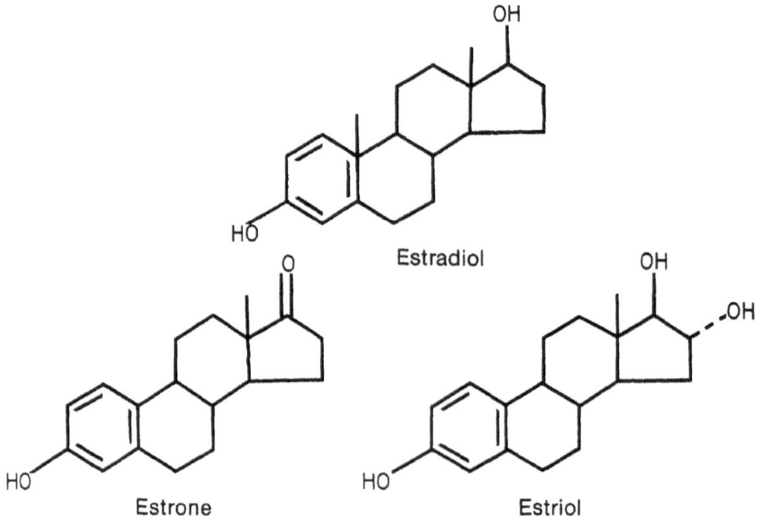

Fig. 11. Structural formulas of the principal natural estrogens

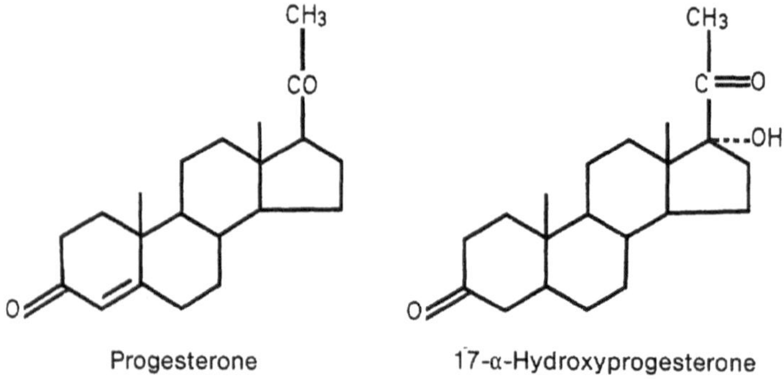

Fig. 12. Structural formulas of the principal natural gestagens

Another pathway which is particularly important in the follicle is that leading from pregnenolone to 17α-hydroxypregnenolone, dehydroepiandrosterone, and finally to androstenedione (Fig. 14).

b) Biologic Effects

Estrogens are compounds which can induce estrus in spayed female rodents. They assure development of the principal female secondary sex characteristics, particularly the typical fat distribution, pelvic shape, and breast development, and aid the adrenocortical androgens in stimulating pubic hair growth. They also promote growth of the genital organs, especially the uterus. Under their influence the vagina lengthens and becomes more distensible. The blood flow to the vulva

10

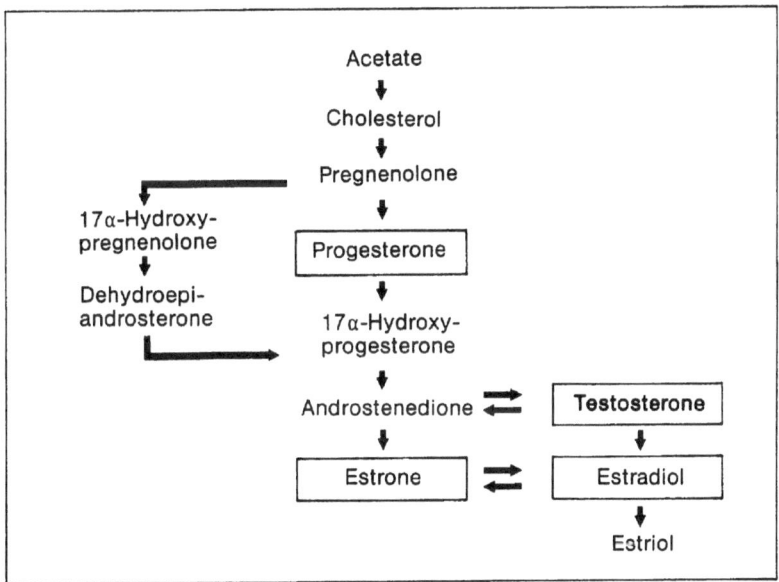

Fig. 13. Structural formulas of the principal natural androgens

Androstendione

Dehydroepiandrosterone

Testosterone

Acetate
↓
Cholesterol
↓
Pregnenolone
↓

17α-Hydroxy-
pregnenolone
↓
Dehydroepi-
androsterone

Progesterone
↓
17α-Hydroxy-
progesterone
↓
Androstenedione ⇄ Testosterone
↓   ↓
Estrone ⇄ Estradiol
↓
Estriol

Fig. 14. Simplified schema of the biosynthesis of sex steroids in the ovary

increases and the labia minora enlarge. The cyclic secretion of estrogens during the reproductive years evokes proliferation of the endometrium, thickening of the vaginal epithelium, and increased permeability of the cervical mucus to sperm (see p 28). The estrogens probably also influence autonomic reactivity by heightening parasympathetic tone. In addition, they cause sodium and water retention and lower the serum cholesterol.

11

Gestagens are steroids whose function is to aid in the development and maintenance of pregnancy. One of their chief functions during the menstrual cycle is to convert the proliferative endometrium into secretory endometrium, thereby preparing the uterus for implantation of a fertilized ovum. If gestagen stimulation is discontinued, withdrawal bleeding results. Together with the estrogens, the gestagens play a major role in breast development: the estrogens stimulate proliferation of the duct system, while the gestagens act mainly on the alveoli. The gestagens also inhibit myometrial contraction, which is particularly important in pregnancy and, like the estrogens, alter the cervical mucus and vaginal epithelium (see p 30). In the autonomic nervous system, they exert a sympathicotonic effect. They promote sodium diuresis but, like the estrogens, cause retention of water. Progesterone, moreover, is thermogenic and produces a rise of 0.4°–0.6° C in body temperature (see p 21).

Androgens are the hormones responsible for the development of male sex characteristics. In females, they are present in small amounts and mainly promote the growth of axillary and pubic hair, as well as development of the clitoris and labia majora. An excess leads to virilization (see p 96). Androgens exert a generally anabolic effect and in higher doses cause a libido increase in women.

3. The Endometrial Cycle

The endometrial cycle can be divided into four main phases: the proliferative phase, the ovulatory phase, the secretory phase, and menstruation. Its average duration is 28 days, ovulation occurring on day 13 or 14 of the cycle.

In the first part of the cycle, the proliferative phase, individual secondary or tertiary follicles mature to Graafian follicles under the action of pituitary gonadotropins, particularly FSH (see p 6). This is accompanied by a progressive increase in ovarian estrogen production (Fig. 15). The functional layers of the endometrium shed during the previous menstruation start to regenerate, and the stroma becomes edematous. The initially narrow, elongated uterine glands, whose epithelia show numerous mitotic figures, grow in from the basal layer (see p 33). The cervical mucus also undergoes characteristic changes as estrogen stimulation increases: it becomes thin, clear, and stretchy and forms fernlike crystals when permitted to dry. Its leukocyte content decreases, while its glucose content and receptivity to sperm increase (see p 28). The vaginal epithelium thickens, glycogen deposits form, and the vaginal smear shows a prevalence of acidophilic superficial cells with pyknotic nuclei.

In the ovulatory phase there is a transitory surge in the secretion of pituitary gonadotropins, especially LH (Fig. 15). Although the central mechanisms which evoke this "midcycle surge" have not been clarified, they most likely involve a positive feedback from the sharply rising estrogen levels and perhaps the 17α-hydroxyprogesterone level, which also rises at this time. A few hours after the LH peak, the mature follicle ruptures and the ovum is discharged.

12

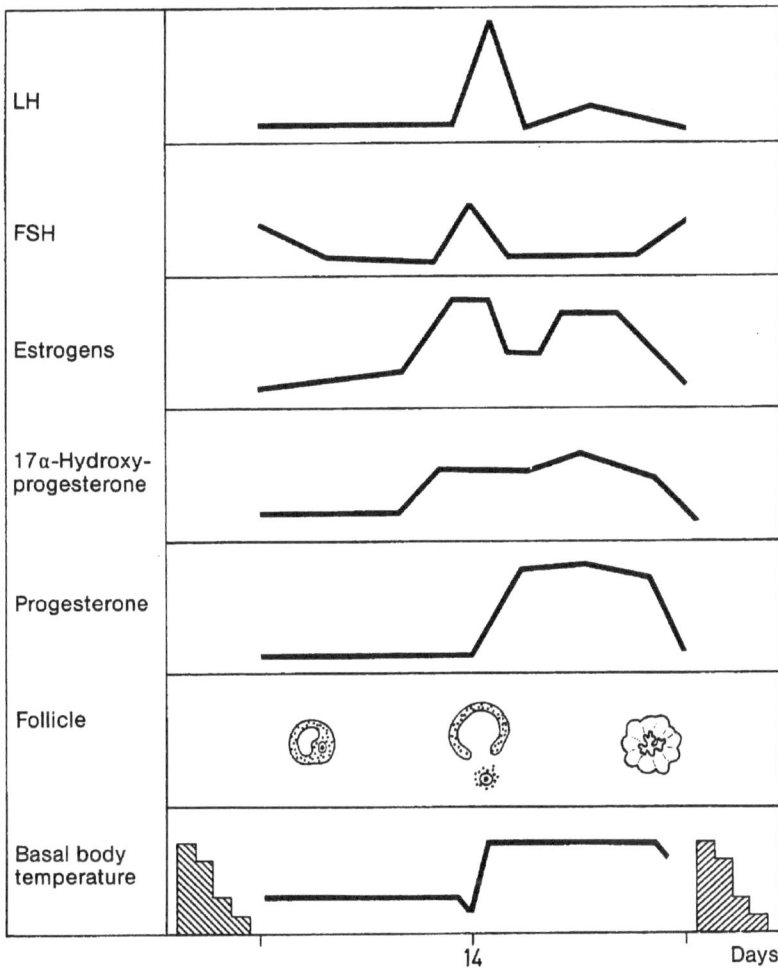

Fig. 15. Schema of hormonal relationships during the normal menstrual cycle

Proliferation of the endometrium is maximal at this time, causing it to attain a thickness of 3 4 mm. The cervical mucus and vaginal epithelium also reflect the strong estrogenic effect.

In the secretory or luteal phase, the postovulatory follicle is transformed into a corpus luteum under the influence of LH. Besides estrogen, the corpus luteum now starts to secrete large amounts of progesterone, which stimulates secretory changes in the endometrium. The glands become tortuous and distended with secretory material as well as glycogen; the epithelial cells show typical retronuclear secretory vacuoles and glycogen deposits. The stroma is highly edematous and is permeated by numerous spiral arterioles. Toward the end of the luteal phase, the glands assume a "sawtoothed" appearance, and pseudodecidual cells appear which closely resemble the decidua of early pregnancy. The cervical mucus decreases in volume under the influence of progesterone. It also becomes cloudy,

13

viscous, and less stretchy. Its leukocyte content increases, and it gradually loses its ability to arborize. The vaginal epithelium undergoes a massive desquamation; the vaginal smear shows a prevalence of clumped, basophilic, intermediate cells (see p 26).

When the corpus luteum ceases its secretory activity, there is a sharp fall in estrogen and progesterone levels. In the endometrium, this causes necrosis, extravasation, and finally, shedding of the functional layers; menstruation has begun. The average blood loss during menstruation is about 80 ml; this blood does not clot readily due to the release of fibrinolytic enzymes. By cycle day 4 or 5, regeneration of the functional layers begins as described above.

III. Conception and Pregnancy

If vital sperm are present in the ampullary portion of the tube at the time of ovulation, fertilization can occur. The life span of the ovum is only about 6–12 h, while the sperm can survive for 2–5 days.

The ovum is exposed to a great number of spermatozoa, but only one succeeds in penetrating the zona pellucida. In the process, the tail of the spermatozoon is lost, while the ovum simultaneously undergoes a second meiosis. During the subsequent conjugation, or fusion of the male and female nuclei, the two sets of haploid chromosomes are combined to form a diploid set of 46 chromosomes. At this moment the development of a new life has begun.

After 30 h the zygote has divided into two cells. After 3 days, it has developed into a morula with about 32 cells. It has also been passively transported by tubal motility into the uterine cavity, where it differentiates into the blastocyst just before implantation (Fig. 16). The blastocyst is a hollow ball of cells consisting of the embryoblast and trophoblast. The former will eventually become the embryo and fetus, while the latter will develop into the placenta. About 6 days after conjugation, the blastocyst implants in the secretory endometrium with the aid of proteolytic enzymes. From this point on, the mother assumes the task of nourishing the embryo. This is the function of the decidua, which develops from the endometrium. The trophoblast differentiates into an inner layer called the cytotrophoblast, which consists of cubic, clearly demarcated cells, and an outer layer called the syncytiotrophoblast, which has indistinct cell boundaries. Implantation is complete 12 days after conception. The epithelium closes, and the primordial villi form. The maternal lacunae dilate to form the intervillous spaces. The villi are supplied with stroma and vessels which later will be involved in embryonic circulation.

Between the 15th and 42nd day after conception, organogenesis takes place within the embryo, with differentiation of the principal organs. During the same period, the definitive placenta is formed as the chorion laeve, i. e., the villous part of the chorion facing the uterine cavity, atrophies, while the chorion frondosum, or the part facing the uterine wall, continues to expand.

14

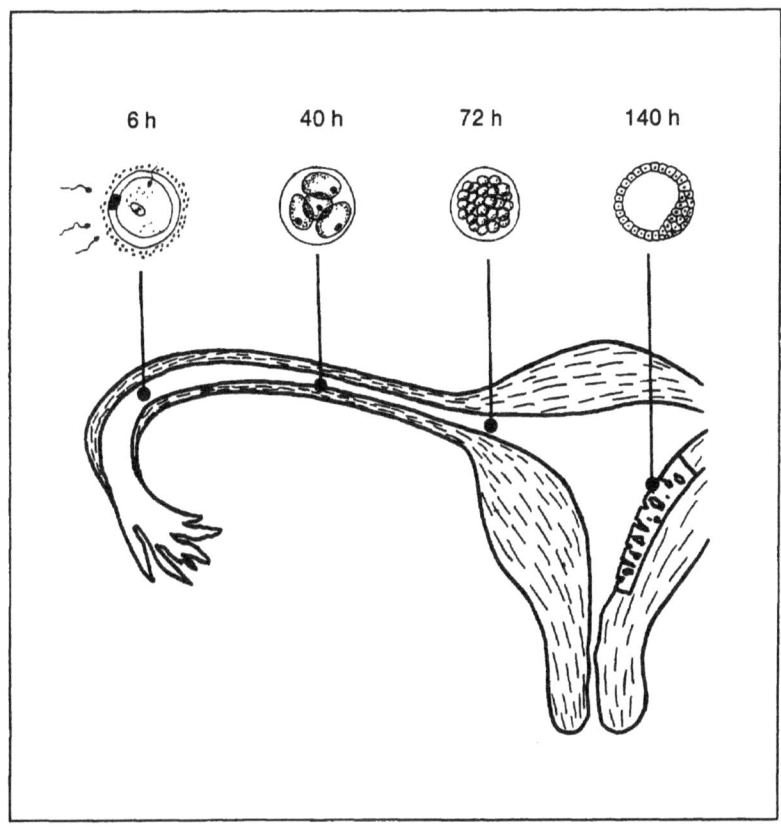

Fig. 16. Schematic representation of the developement of the fertilized ovum and its transport

In many cases this process is interrupted prematurely by spontaneous abortion, and often the fertilized ovum fails even to implant. Extensive studies have shown that 50% of unimplanted ova display malformations which render them incapable of normal development. Even after implantation has occurred, about one-third of pregnancies still terminate in early abortion, frequently unnoticed by the woman. With regard to the endocrine system, pregnancy is characterized by significant hormonal shifts. After about 10 days' gestation the trophoblast starts to secrete a new hormone, human chorionic gonadotropin (HCG). Owing to its strong luteotropic action, it prevents regression of the corpus luteum, converting it instead into the corpus luteum of pregnancy, which secretes increasing amounts of estrogens and progesterone. These hormones prevent the menstrual breakdown of the endometrium and promote its conversion into the decidua. Afterwards, this function is increasingly assumed by the large amounts of steroid hormones produced by the trophoblast itself. These steroids are essential for the development and maintenance of pregnancy, as well as for the later preparation for parturition. Under their influence the pituitary production of gonadotropins ceases almost completely for the duration of the pregnancy, to gradually resume only after postpartum expulsion of the placenta.

The further development of the pregnancy and the endocrine relations between the mother, placenta, and fetus, as well as the special hormonal aspects of parturition and lactation are quite complex and beyond the scope of this book.

IV. Puberty, the Climacteric and the Postmenopause Period

1. Puberty

The ovaries are almost completely inactive until prepuberty, which occurs at about the age of 8 or 9. At this time the pituitary begins to secrete gonadotropins secondary to the suspension of certain central inhibitory mechanisms which are still poorly understood. These hormones stimulate the ovary to produce significant amounts of estrogens for the first time. Under their influence the uterus enlarges, the corpus increasing in size more than the cervix. The first outward pubertal sign, occurring at age 10 or 11, is the development of breast buds – the thelarche. True puberty begins a short time later with the appearance of pubic hair. This results from an increase in the production of adrenal steroids, which are probably also responsible for the pubertal growth spurt. A year or two after the pubarche, axillary hair appears. Also at this time the estrogens stimulate further development of the vagina and labia minora and cause the pelvis to acquire its characteristic female shape.

The most striking pubertal event is the occurrence of the first menstruation, called the menarche. In Central Europe the menarche occurs at about age 13 on the average (Fig. 17a). It appears before age 9 or after age 16 in only about 5% of girls. The first menstruation is usually anovular and is the result of estrogen withdrawal. Ovulatory cycles occur with increasing frequency during the adolescent phase, which lasts until the completion of growth. Fertility is low at first but increases rapidly. The initial menstrual cycles are highly irregular, and dysfunctional bleeding is common (see p 68).

2. The Climacteric

The climacteric is a term describing the span of several years before and after the menopause, the time at which menstruation ceases. More precisely, the climacteric can be divided into the premenopausal and postmenopausal phase.

The premenopausal phase begins 2–3 years before the menopause and is characterized by a gradual decline of ovarian estrogen production. Central control becomes increasingly erratic and cyclic gonadotropin release increasingly irregular.

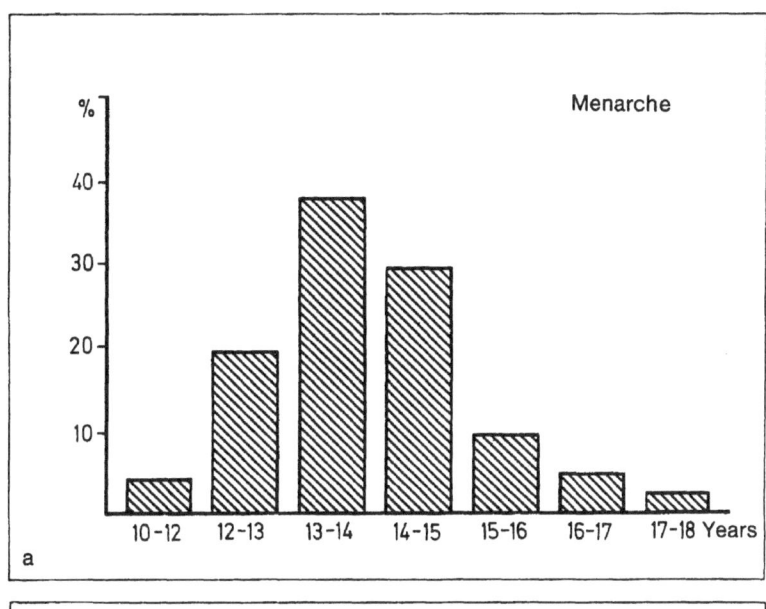

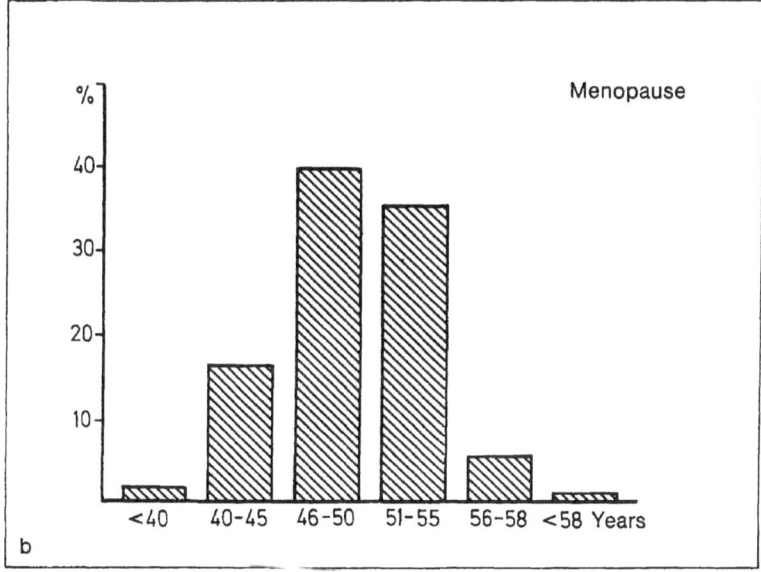

Fig. 17. a Percentage incidence of the onset of menarche by age group. **b** Percentage incidence of the onset of menopause by age group

Menstrual irregularities and dysfunctional bleeding (see p 93) are frequent. As the ovaries become less responsive to pituitary stimuli, there is a gradual compensatory rise of gonadotropin levels, which can maintain a marginal degree of ovarian function for some time. However, fertility is low and pregnancy rarely occurs. When estrogen production decreases further and excretory values fall below about 10 μg/24 h, menstrual bleeding ceases completely. This event, the menopause, occurs at an average age of 52 at European latitudes (Fig. 17b), although there are wide variations. Nevertheless, only about 5% of women experience menopause before age 40 or after age 58.

During the postmenopausal phase that follows, there is a further increase in gonadotropin secretion. The FSH levels, in particular, are 5–20 times higher than during the reproductive years. Although the ovaries still contain a small number of primary follicles, their response to pituitary stimulation is extremely weak or absent. The resulting estrogen deficiency is responsible for the "menopausal syndrome," characterized by flushing and a variety of other objective and subjective symptoms (see p 92). The endometrium shows some signs of proliferation for a few more years; the vaginal epithelium also shows evidence of an estrogenic effect for several years after the menopause.

By 6 to 8 years after the menopause, the genital organs have undergone pronounced involutional changes, marking the start of the senium.

V. Importance of Endocrine Interactions

Female sexual function is strongly dependent on hormonal sources other than the sex-specific endocrine systems. One important source is the adrenal cortex, which produces a number of steroids under the influence of pituitary adrenocorticotropic hormone (ACTH). Foremost among the adrenocortical steroids are the mineralocorticoids, such as aldosterone and desoxycorticosterone, which are mainly concerned with regulating sodium and potassium metabolism as well as water balance. The glucocorticoids cortisone and corticosterone act mainly on sugar metabolism by increasing gluconeogenesis, but also influence protein and lipid metabolism. Additionally, the adrenal cortex produces a number of sex steroids, chiefly androgens, and thus figures prominently in the development of certain secondary sex characteristics, such as the growth of genital and axillary hair.

Adrenocortical dysfunction has adverse effects on both the menstrual cycle and fertility (see p 97), as do other endocrine disorders, especially those involving the pituitary. Of particular importance is the oversecretion of prolactin, which leads to amenorrhea and sterility (see p 85), probably by a direct inhibition of follicle maturation and ovulation. Finally, the more severe forms of hypo- and hyperthyroidism can also cause menstrual disturbances.

B. Diagnosis of Hormonal Disorders

I. Basic Principles

Hormonal disorders are not only very frequent in gynecology, but are also very distressful to the patient due to the sterility that often results. For these reasons it is important in gynecology, as in medicine generally, to obtain as much information as possible using simple diagnostic methods and then to institute specific treatment.

In this chapter we discuss the most important methods currently used for the investigation of menstrual disorders, infertility, and virilism. The diagnostic program must necessarily be individualized, although a few purely clinical tests will often suffice for practical purposes. In cases of amenorrhea, an accurate diagnosis can be made on the basis of the basal temperature curve, gestagen test, and pituitary gonadotropin assay. In hirsutism, anamnesis, general findings, and testosterone assay may be sufficient to determine etiology. On the other hand, conditions such as virilism or unexplained sterility may necessitate very intensive investigative procedures. Such cases should be identified early and referred to a specialist.

II. Clinical Aspects

1. Anamnesis

Anamnesis plays a key role in the investigation of hormonal disorders in gynecology. Besides the usual questions, special attention is given to the course of puberty, the age of menarche, thelarche, adrenarche (pubarche), and the menstrual cycle with regard to the rhythm, duration, and amount of menstrual bleeding. This will reveal any preexisting menstrual irregularities.

The patient is then questioned about inter-, pre-, and postmenstrual bleeding, as well as dysmenorrhea, premenstrual complaints, and discharge. Parous women should be asked about the course of their pregnancy, the delivery, and the lactation period, since some endocrinopathies such as Sheehan's syndrome (see p 86) are directly associated with parturition. Also important are weight changes, which are typical of Cushing's syndrome and anorexia nervosa, voice changes, and hirsutism in virilization, as well as the presence of flushes in premature menopause (see p 86) or headaches and visual disturbances in pituitary tumors. Finally, since menstrual dysfunction is sometimes of psychological origin, the physician should examine the patient's relationships to her marital or sexual partner, school, home, or place of employment. These factors are particularly important in women with secondary amenorrhea.

2. Clinical Examination

The general examination also provides much useful information. Besides the physical appearance and physique, weight, and size, particular attention is given to the development of secondary sex characteristics, the breasts and body hair. In many diseases, such as marked hypogonadism, gonadal dysgenesis, testicular feminization, anorexia nervosa, or Sheehan's syndrome, a diagnosis is suggested almost at once by the clinical picture (see Figs. 67, 68, 69, 71, 79).

The examiner should also be alert for signs of disorders of other endocrine glands, particularly the thyroid, adrenal cortex, and anterior pituitary; associated symptoms include goiter, exophthalmos, a cushingoid aspect, virilization, galactorrhea, and acromegaly.

3. Gynecologic Examination

The gynecologic exploration is undertaken in the usual manner, though extra tact is required due to the sensitiveness of many of these patients. The external genitalia are first evaluated for their development, special note being made of the clitoris, which is enlarged in virilization; the labia minora, which generally are underdeveloped in hypogonadism; and the genital hair, which may be feminine, sparse, or virile, depending on the endocrine status.

The speculum examination gives information on the presence of a vagina, the vaginal contents, the size of the portio, and the character of the cervical mucus (see p 28), which in turn may be suggestive of ovarian failure.

Finally, bimanual examination is done to assess the shape and size of the uterus. The adnexal regions in particular are carefully palpated. Ovarian enlargement is found in the Stein-Leventhal syndrome (see p 87) or may be secondary to a hormone-producing tumor.

III. Special Investigations

1. Basal Body Temperature

Measurement of the basal body temperature (BBT) is a simple, generally applicable method of evaluating the menstrual cycle. The patient is instructed to take her temperature rectally at about the same time each morning immediately upon waking, preferably after at least 6 h rest. The same thermometer must be used for all measurements; special models with a large, easy-to-read scale, such as the "Cyclotest," are best suited for this purpose. The thermometer should be held in the rectum for 5 min and the readings entered on a special chart (Fig. 18). Any unusual circumstances that might influence the temperature curve (such as over-sleeping, malaise, or infection) should be noted. In sterility cases, acts of inter-course are also recorded. Experience has shown that adequate patient instruction is mandatory. The curves are sometimes useless because the thermometer was not shaken down before use or was not properly placed in the rectum.

The basal body temperature is a very good index of hormonal processes. After menstruation and throughout the proliferative phase of the cycle, it ranges from 36.3° to 36.8°C. At ovulation, the temperature is at a low point in many women. The basal temperature rises 1–2 days later by 0.4°–0.7°C owing to the ther-mogenic effect of ovarian progesterone secretion; it then measures 36.9°–37.4°C until shortly before menstruation. This "hyperthermal plateau" normally lasts 10–14 days (Fig. 19).

There are characteristic deviations from this normal pattern which are easily re-cognized. First, the basal temperature curve recorded over a period of months may show a monophasic course, i. e., the midcycle thermal shift is absent. This usually indicates failure of ovulation and thus the absence of corpus luteum formation (Fig. 20). But this is not necessarily the case, since the curve may be monophasic even if a normal, progesterone-secreting corpus luteum is present. Another devia-tion is a shortening of the hyperthermal plateau to less than 10 days; moreover, the thermal shift may take place gradually over a period of 3–6 days, rather than the usual 1–2 (Fig. 21 a, b). Both patterns are indicative of inadequate corpus

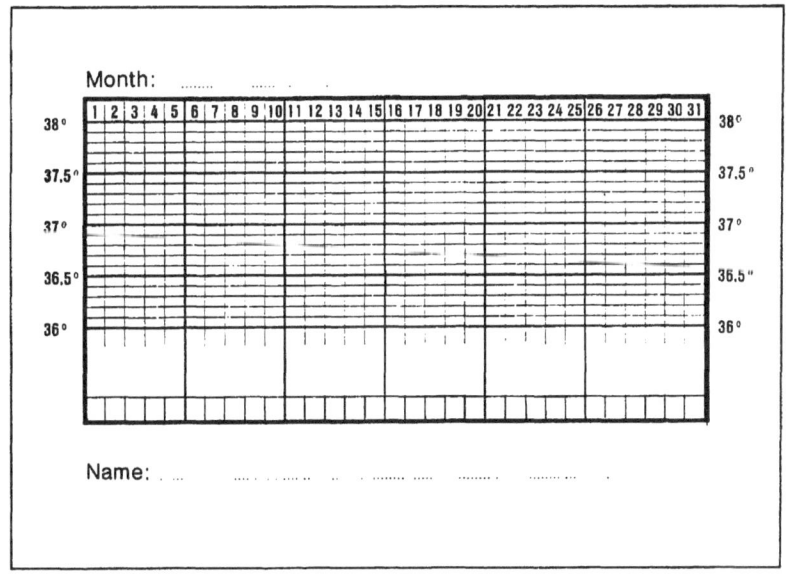

Fig. 18. Chart for recording the basal body temperature

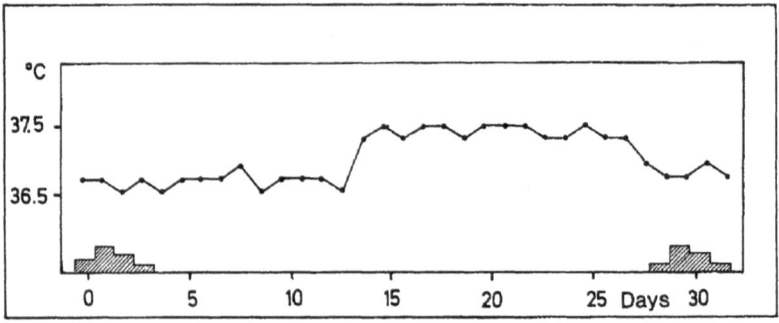

Fig. 19. Basal temperature record of normal cycle

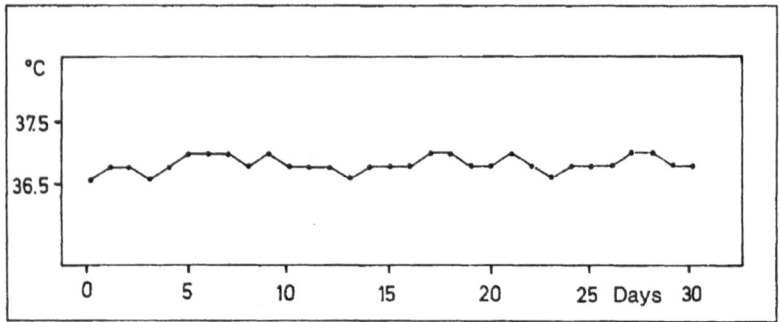

Fig. 20. Basal temperature record of anovulatory cycle

luteum function, or "luteal phase insufficiency" which leads to sterility. The basal body temperature may also remain elevated for a prolonged period. A hyperthermal plateau lasting more than 16 days after a corresponding rise is a reliable indication of early pregnancy (Fig. 22), long before commercial pregnancy tests give a positive result.

The basal temperature curve is also useful in sterility cases as a means of determining the fertility peak – a reverse form of the Knaus-Ogino method. Accordingly, the best time for intercourse is just before the rise of the basal body temperature, in the region of the low point, if present. This is particularly important for the timing of artificial insemination.

2. Vaginal Cytology

The microscopic appearance of the vaginal cells is an accurate indicator of hormonal processes and thus offers a highly useful, simple and inexpensive means of assessing menstrual function. A speculum is inserted, and cellular material is removed from the lateral fornix with a cotton swab. It is immediately spread with a rolling motion onto a clean glass slide and fixed in 1:1 ether-alcohol (96%) for at

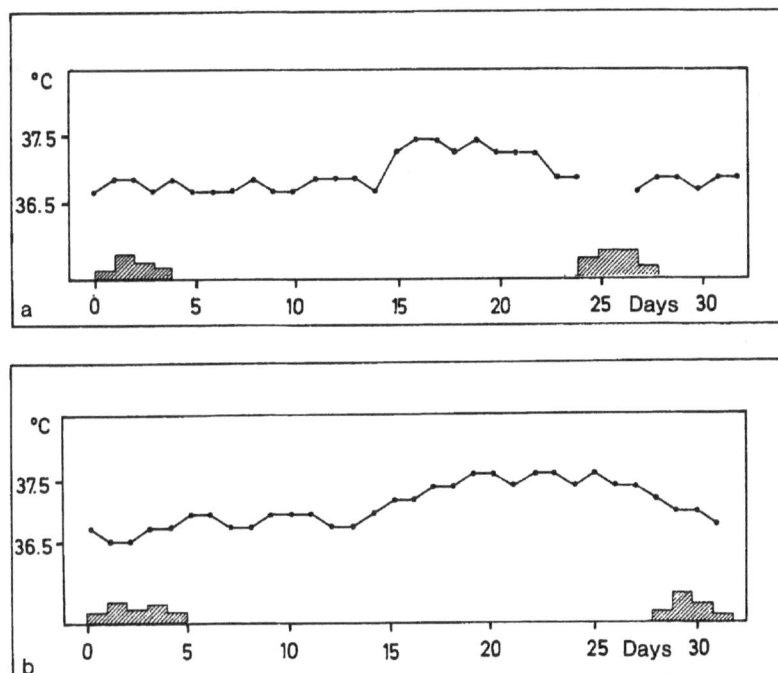

Fig. 21. a Basal temperature record of luteal inadequacy with shortened hyperthermal plateau. **b** Basal temperature record of luteal deficiency with prolonged "staircase" thermal shift

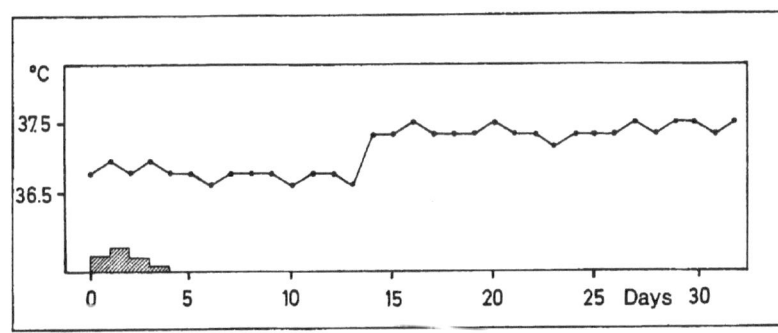

Fig. 22. Basal temperature record of early pregnancy

least 30 min. A spray fixative such as Merckofix or Spray-Cyto (Adams) may be used for this purpose. The smear is stained by the method of Shorr or Papanicolaou (Table 1), as is customary in every cytology laboratory. With experience, the evaluation can be made by direct examination with a phase-contrast microscope.

Interpretation of the exfoliative cytologic picture requires a certain basic knowledge of the structure and hormonal response of the vaginal epithelium (Figs. 23,

Table 1. Procedure for staining of vaginal smears (modified from Papanicolaou)

1. 5 min 80% isopropyl alcohol
2. 2 min Harris' hematoxylin (Merck)
3. 1 min running water
4. 3 min orange G solution (Merck)
5. 1 min 80% isopropyl alcohol
6. 2 min polychrome solution EA 50 (Merck)
7. 1 min 80% isopropyl alcohol
8. 1 min 95% isopropyl alcohol
9. 3 min absol. isopropyl alcohol – xylene (4:3)
10. 5 min xylene
11. 5 min xylene

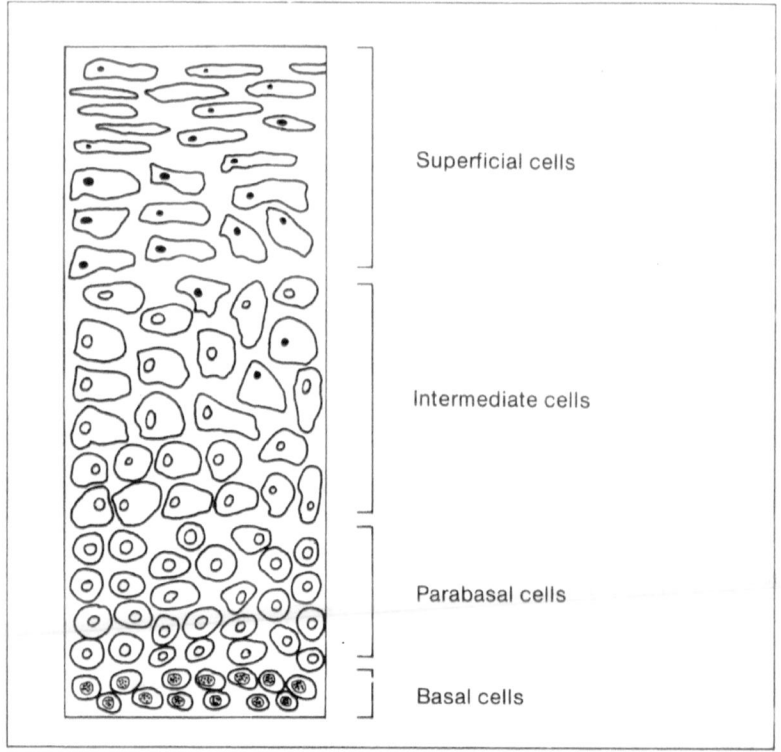

Fig. 23. Schematic structure of the vaginal epithelium

24). Basically, four layers can be distinguished: superficial, intermediate, parabasal, and basal. Accordingly, four main cell types are found in the vaginal secretion after exfoliation. Superficial cells are large and polygonal, their nuclei are often pyknotic, and the cytoplasm may be acidophilic or basophilic, depending on the phase of the cycle. The smaller, ovoid intermediate cells have vesicular nuclei, and their cytoplasm is basophilic on staining. Parabasal cells are small, circular,

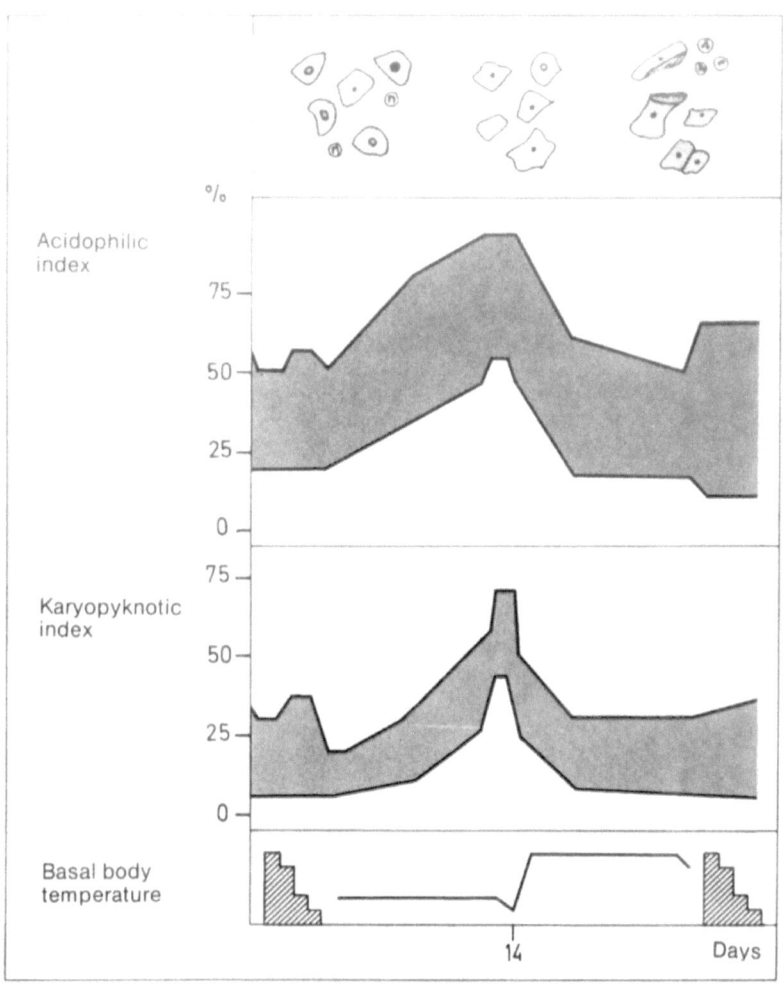

Fig. 24. Acidophilic and karyopyknotic index of vaginal smear in a normal cycle

and basophilic with large, chromatin-rich nuclei. The basal cells are the smallest and have the most prominent nuclei. Two important quantitative measures of vaginal cell status are the pyknotic index, which is the percentage of superficial cells with pyknotic nuclei, and the acidophilic index, which is the percentage of superficial cells with acidophilic cytoplasm.

During the course of the menstrual cycle, the cytologic picture undergoes characteristic changes (Fig. 24). The early follicular phase is marked by an increasing number of superficial cells in relation to intermediate cells. They are still mainly basophilic, and only some of their nuclei are pyknotic. At this time the pyknotic index is 30%–60%, the acidophilic index about 30% (Fig. 25). As ovulation approaches, there is an increasing prevalence of superficial cells. At ovulation, when the estrogenic effect is maximal, the cells are almost entirely of the superficial type with strongly pyknotic nuclei. The pyknotic index may increase to 90%,

25

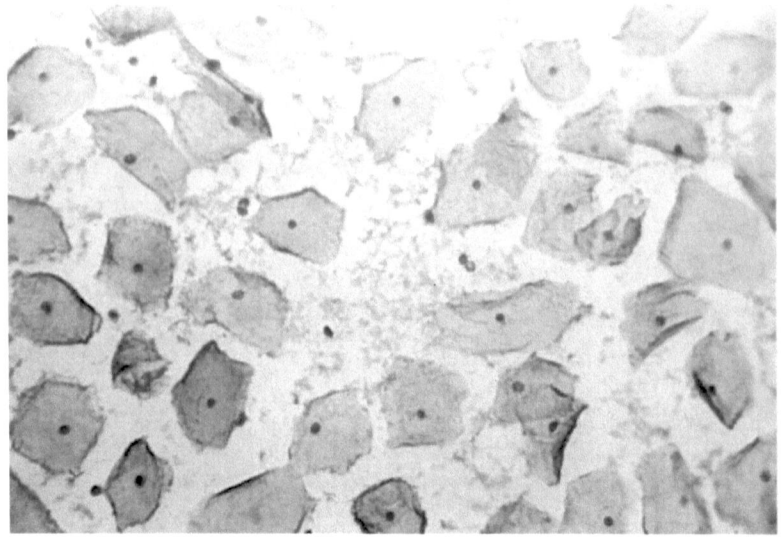

Fig. 25. Vaginal smear in the early proliferative phase: basophilic superficial and intermediate cells (x 250)

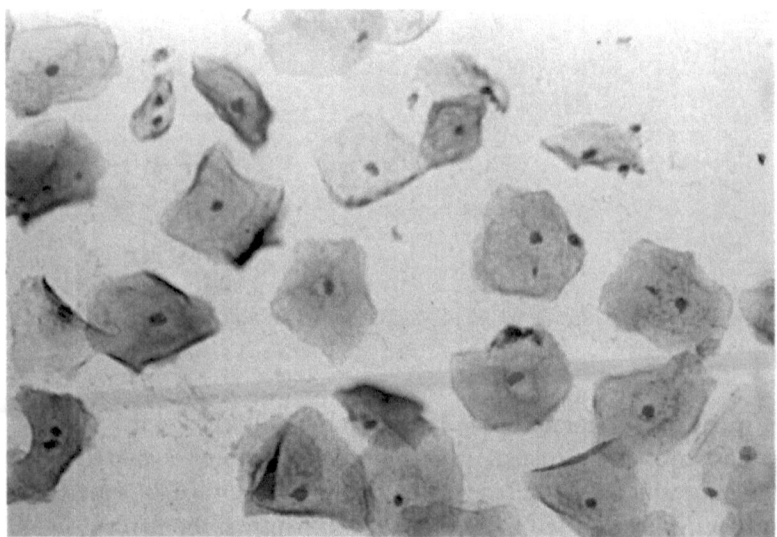

Fig. 26

the acidophilic index to 70% (Fig. 26). At the same time, the previously abundant leukocytes are completely absent. In the luteal phase, the picture is modified by the addition of progesteronic effects. The superficial cells become increasingly basophilic and folded, clumping occurs, the pyknotic and acidophilic indexes fall below 30%, and increasing numbers of leukocytes appear (Fig. 27). Basophilic,

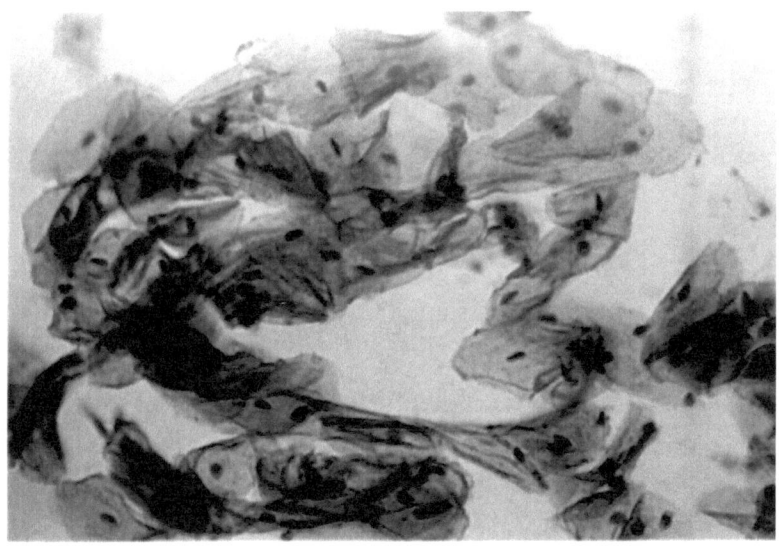

Fig. 27. Vaginal smear in the secretory phase: partially clumped, basophilic intermediate cells with curled edges (x 250)

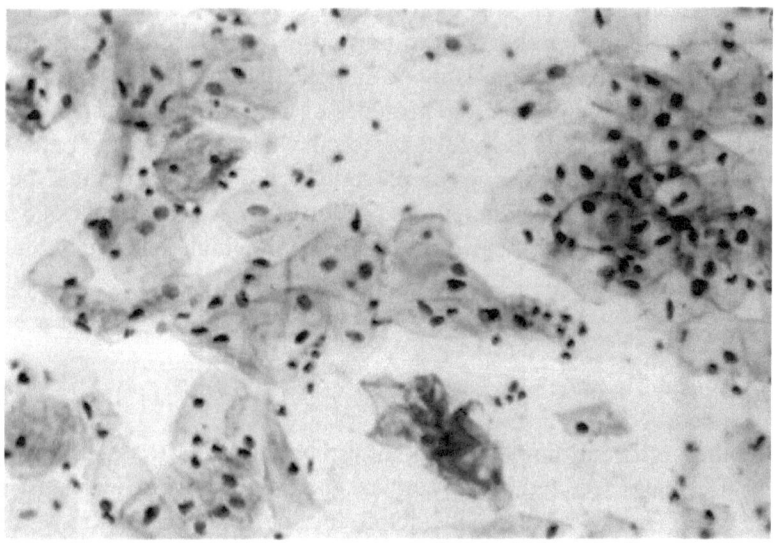

Fig. 28. Vaginal smear in pregnancy: navicular cells (x 250)

folded superficial cells also occur in pregnancy, but the "navicular cells" from the intermediate layer are predominant in the later course (Fig. 28).

"Atrophic" smears with predominantly basal and parabasal cells and some intermediate cells (Fig. 29) are characteristic of children and postmenopausal women, as well as women with marked ovarian failure. During the transitional phases, i. e., puberty and the climacteric phase, the picture can vary greatly depending on the

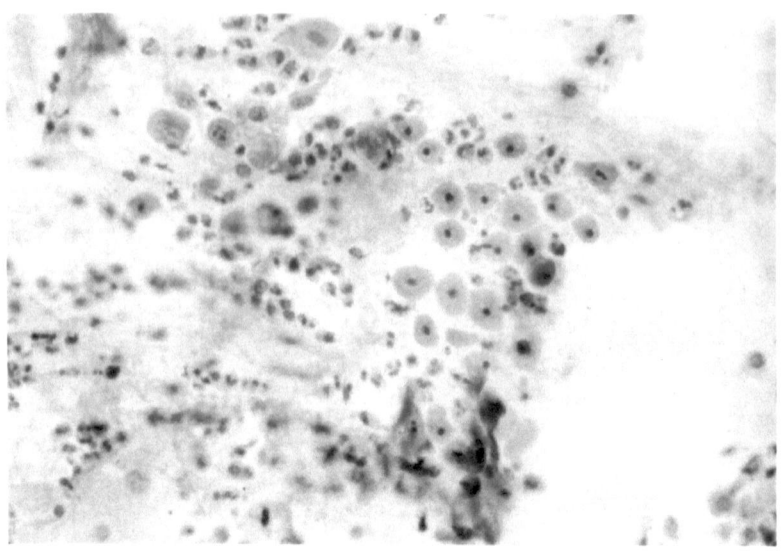

Fig. 29. "Atrophic" vaginal smear after menopause: parabasal and basal cells, leukocytes (x 250)

hormonal situation; thus, an estrogenic effect with the corresponding signs may be demonstrable in prepuberty as well as up to 2 years after menopause.

Hormonal vaginal cytology may be complicated by various factors. For example, interpretation is vitiated in the presence of inflammation. In such cases a terramycin suppository should be inserted into the vagina several days before the smear is obtained. As in all diagnostic procedures, of course, it must be determined whether the patient has taken medication such as oral contraceptives and other hormonal preparations, since the vaginal epithelium is strongly affected by synthetic sex steroids.

3. Cervical Mucus

Another rapid and simple method of estimating the hormonal status is by evaluating the mucus secreted by the cervical glands (Fig. 30). After menstruation, when the external cervical os is constricted, the sparse mucus is cloudy, tacky, viscous, and impermeable to sperm (see p 40). As the estrogen level rises, the mucus increases in quantity and becomes more transparent, thinner, and more elastic. Finally, at ovulation, it flows in copious amounts from the dilated external os (Fig. 31); it is clear, stretchy, and optimally receptive to sperm. With the post-ovulatory rise of progesterone, these changes regress and the mucus again becomes scanty and opaque.

The effect of estrogen on the cervical mucus is particularly evident in the thread-like quality, or *spinnbarkeit,* of the mucus. This can be tested by taking some mucus from the cervical canal with a dissecting forceps and stretching it between

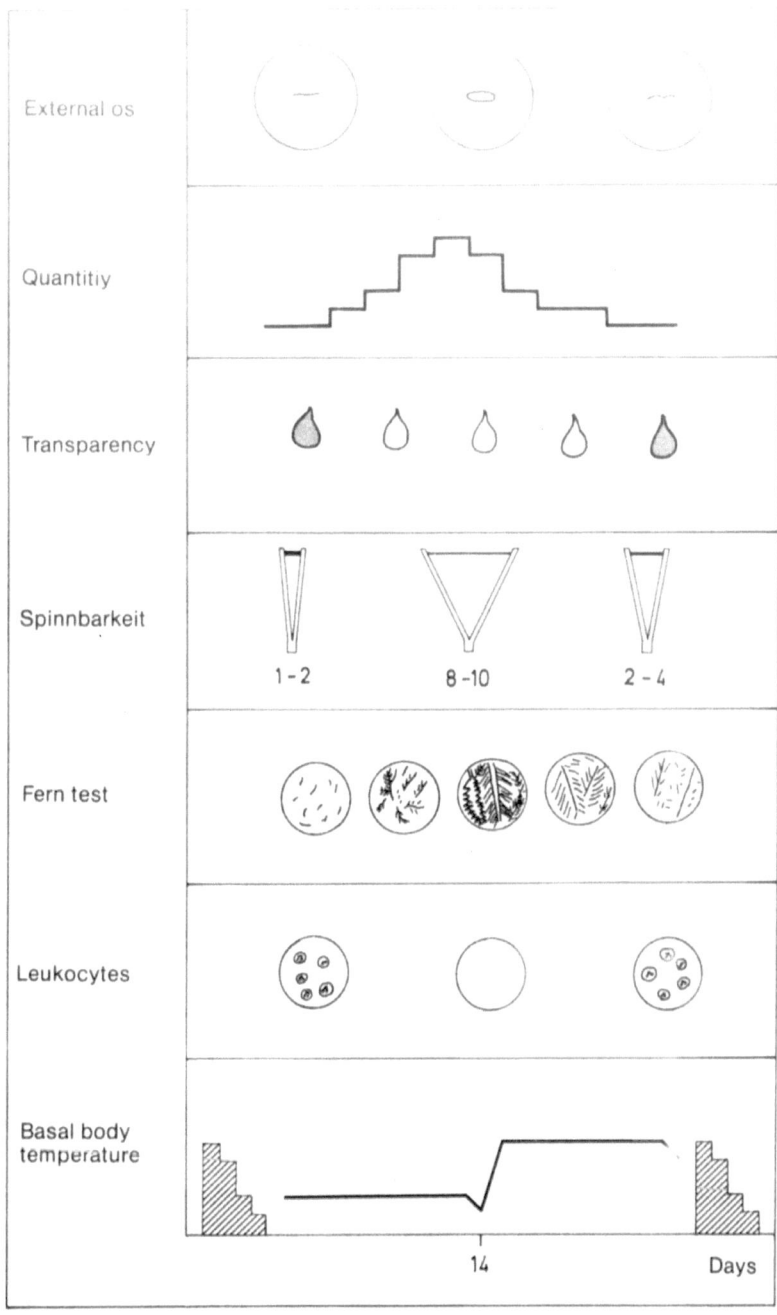

Fig. 30. Changes in the external os and cervical mucus during the normal cycle

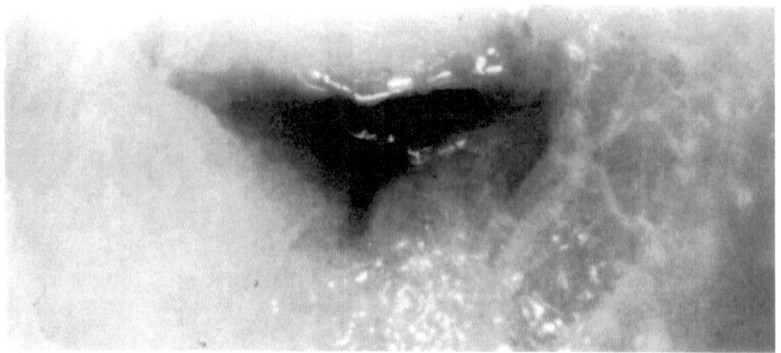

Fig. 31. Dilated external os with abundant clear mucus at the time of ovulation

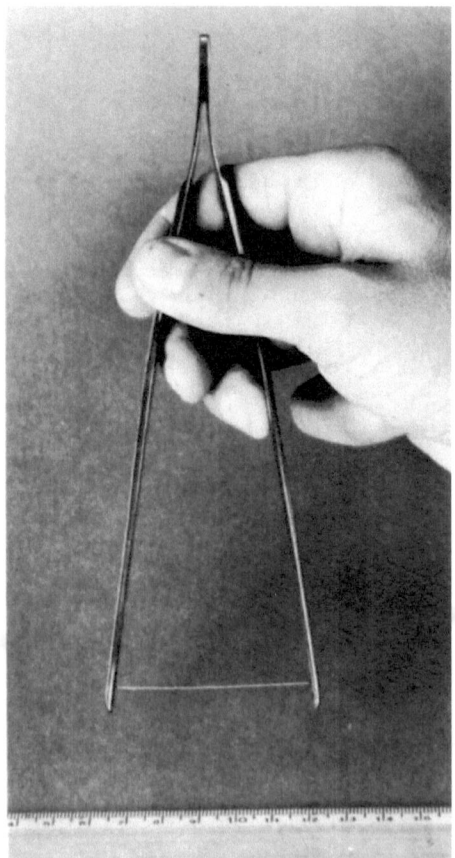

Fig. 32. Test for the *spinnbarkeit* of cervical mucus

the forceps jaws. At ovulation the mucus can be stretched into a thread 6–12 cm long (Fig. 32). At the onset of the proliferative phase and under the influence of progesterone during the second half of the cycle, the *spinnbarkeit* decreases to 0–2 cm. Low *spinnbarkeit* is also typical of ovarian failure and the postmenopausal period.

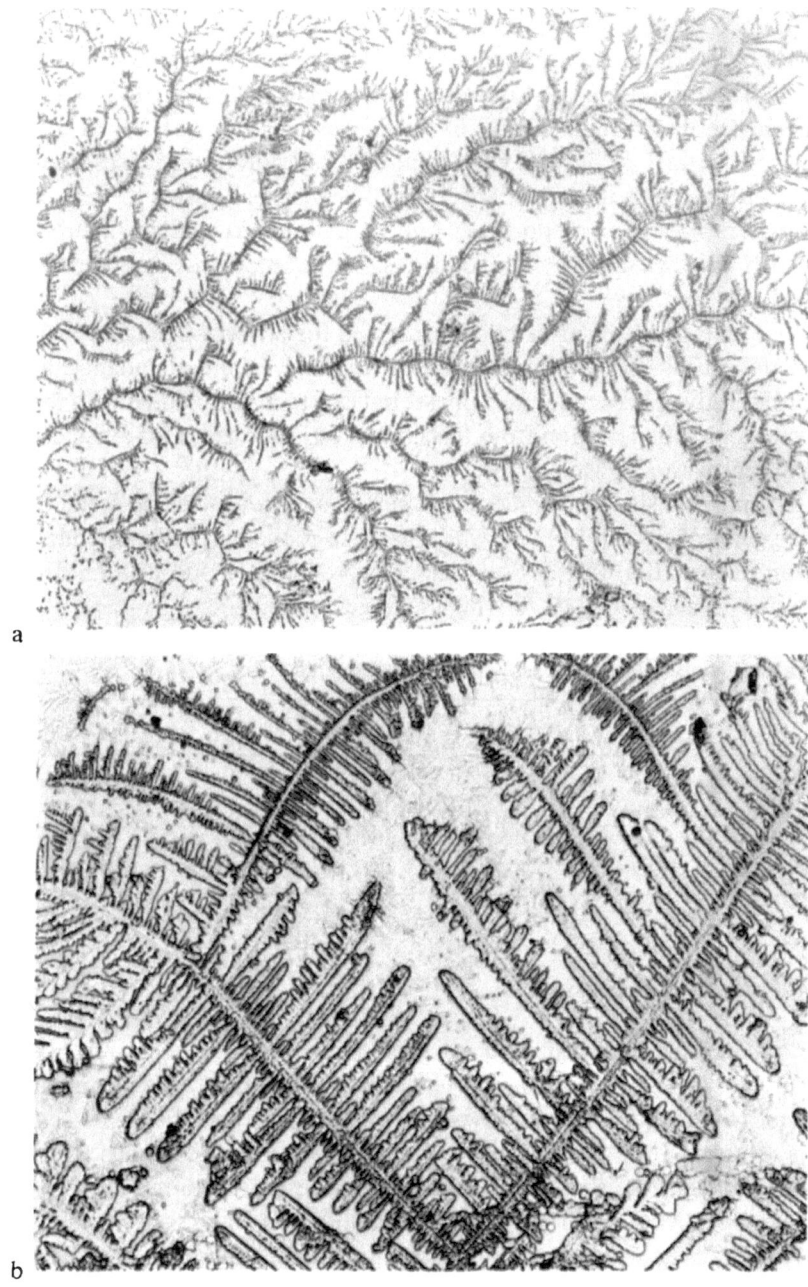

Fig. 33. a Weakly positive fern test during moderate estrogen activity in the early proliferative phase. **b** Strongly positive fern test during maximal estrogen activity at time of ovulation

31

Another method of evaluating the cervical mucus is the "fern test". A small amount of mucus is placed on a clean glass slide, left uncovered, and permitted to dry. In the presence of strong estrogenic activity, striking "fern-leaf" crystals will form due to the high salinity of the mucus (Fig. 33 a, b). When the influence of estrogen starts to decline while that of progesterone increases, the arborization pattern becomes ill-defined. It is completely absent during the pre- and postmenstrual phase, after menopause, and in autonomic ovarian failure. Clean slides which have not come in contact with saline solution are essential, of course, for an accurate fern test.

While the dried mucus is being examined for arborization, the leukocyte content of the mucus should also be assessed. Leukocytes are abundant during the early proliferative phase and luteal phase, but sparse at ovulation due to the influence of estrogen. Any deviation from this pattern is justification for a bacteriologic study, perhaps with a resistance test.

A comprehensive assessment of all factors mentioned can be made on the basis of the cervical score (Table 2), which has also proved useful in optimizing the induction of ovulation (see p 84). Values of 4–7 correspond to a moderate estrogen activity, values of 8–12 to a high estrogen activity.

Table 2. Cervical score in assessment of estrogenic effect

	0	1	2	3
Quantity	–	+	+ +	+ + +
Spinnbarkeit (cm)	0	1–2	3–7	8–10
Fern test	Amorphous	Linear	Partial	Complete
External os	Closed		Partially open	Gaping

4. Endometrial Biopsy

Endometrial biopsy can be done as an office procedure using a small endometrial curet or Novak suction curet. The cervix and vagina are thoroughly disinfected, the cavity length is measured with a hysterometer, and the desired strip of mucosa is removed from the anterior or posterior wall of the fundus. Dilatation of the cervical canal is usually unnecessary; anesthesia is required only in special cases. The specimen is fixed in 96% alcohol, and a special glycogen stain is advantageous. The histologic interpretation requires some experience. The main purpose of this biopsy is to check for secretory changes in the endometrium (see p 13) if anovulation or luteal inadequacy is suspected. It should be performed in all cases of sterility with a short hyperthermal phase, preferably 7–10 days after the midcycle shift. At this time the normal endometrial specimen shows dilated, "sawtooth" glands containing mucus and glycogen, an edematous stroma, and spiral arterioles (Fig. 34). If ovulation has failed to occur, with a consequent progesterone deficiency, the endometrium is of the proliferative type with elongated or somewhat tortuous glands devoid of glycogen (Fig. 35). In autonomic ovarian failure with an

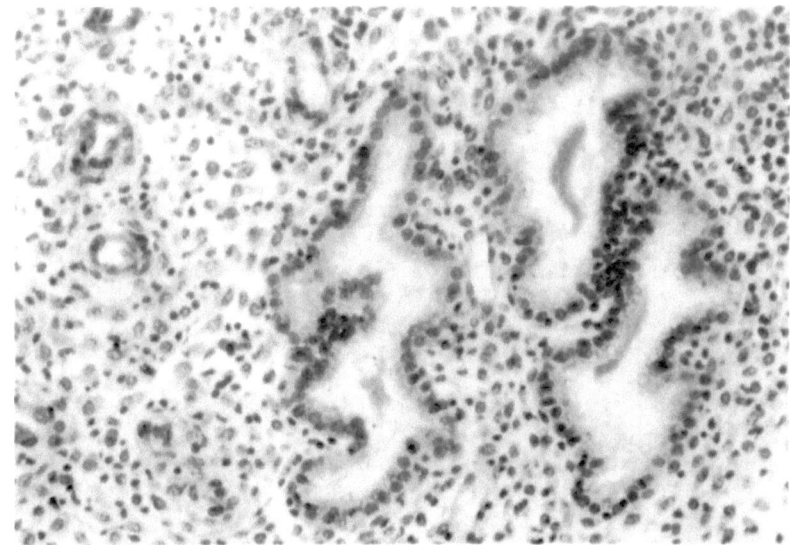

Fig. 34. Endometrium in the sectretory phase, 10 days after ovulation (x 60)

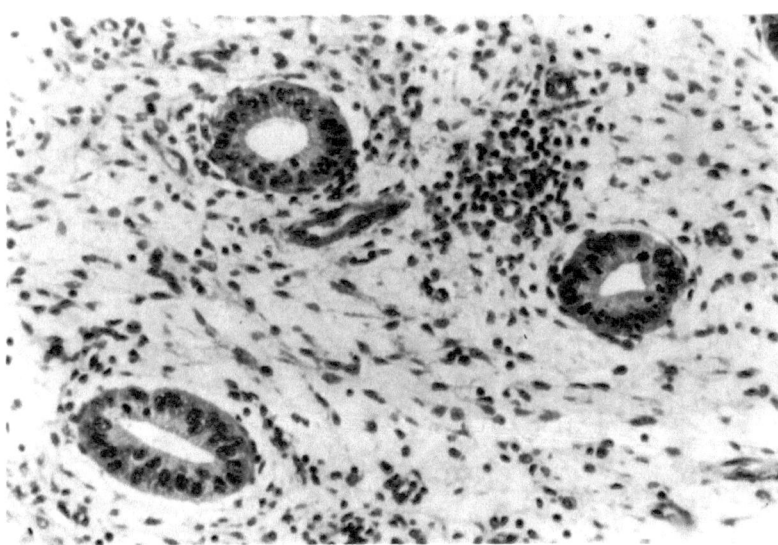

Fig. 35. Endometrium in the proliferative phase (x 60)

absence of follicle maturation and estrogen secretion, the endometrium is quiescent to atropic (Fig. 36).

5. Chromosomal Sex Determination

A chromosomal sex determination is performed in cases of primary amenorrhea, certain cases of virilization, and genital malformations. The simplest method is to search for the sex chromatin in cells from a buccal smear or from the hair root. In

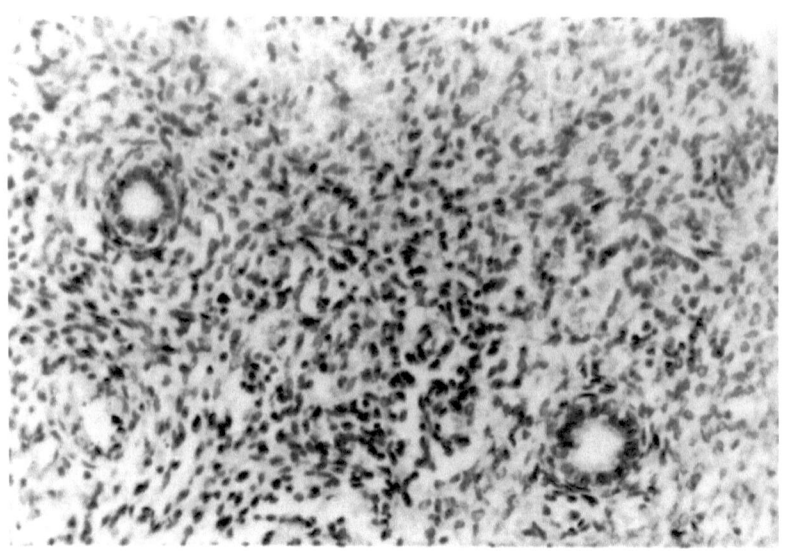

Fig. 36. Atrophic endometrium in marked estrogen deficiency (x 60)

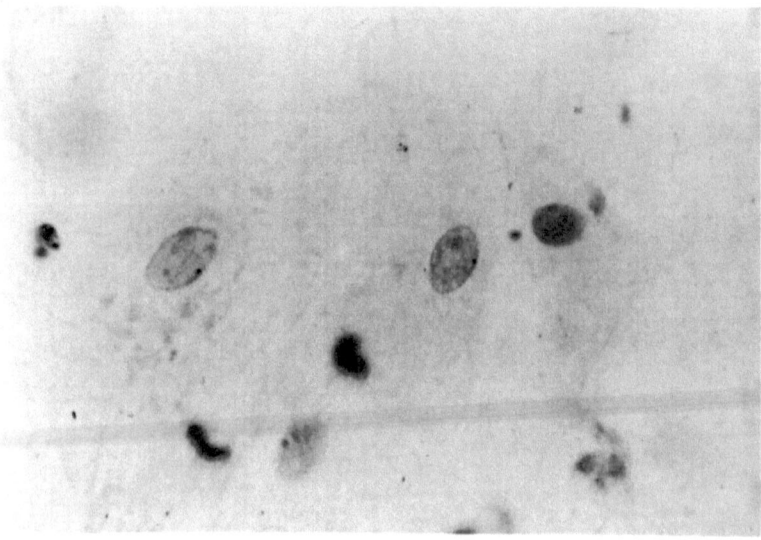

Fig. 37. Determination of chromosomal sex from buccal smear; presence of chromatin bodies indicates genetic female

the female, with two X chromosomes, a chromatin mass adjacent to the inner surface of the nuclear membrane is observed in over 30% of the cell nuclei; this mass corresponds to the second, genetically inactive X chromosome. In the male, with an XY chromosome set, this mass is largely absent (Fig. 37).
Analogously, a drumstick-like structure about 1.5 μ in diameter is found in 2%–3% of the neutrophilic leukocytes in the blood smear of the female (Fig. 38);

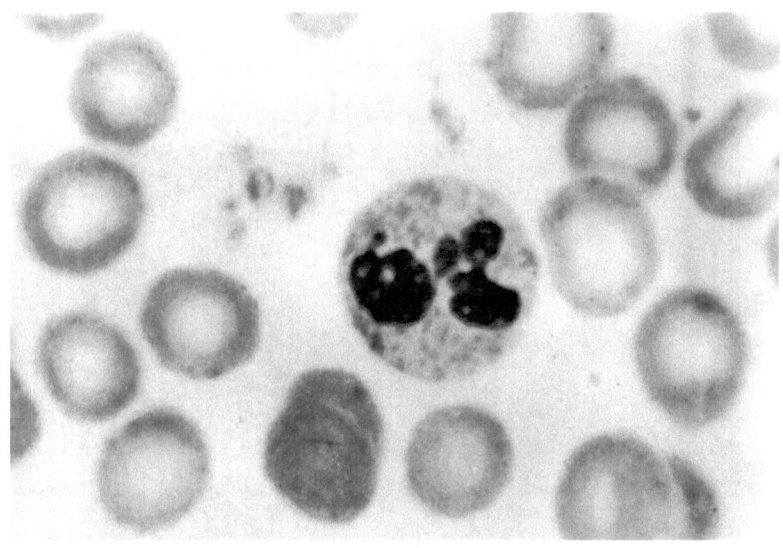

Fig. 38. Determination of chromosomal sex from blood smear; presence of drumsticks in neutrophils indicates female

the drumstick is not present in the male. When more detailed genetic information is required, a complete chromosome analysis must be carried out. But this requires special laboratory facilities and so is reserved for special cases.

6. Laparoscopy

Laparoscopy is today probably the best method for simultaneously evaluating the uterus, tubes, and ovaries with a minimal degree of difficulty (Fig. 39a). It may be done under local anesthesia, but general anesthesia is preferred. After a pneumoperitoneum is created by insufflation of CO_2, the laparoscope is introduced subumbilically. The internal genital organs are systematically localized. Tubal patency can be simultaneously checked by the transuterine injection of dilute sterile indigo carmine using a salpingographic cannula (Fig. 39b).

Purely diagnostic laparoscopy is a low-risk procedure but, of course, is not recommended following a previous laparotomy with adhesions. In the diagnosis of hormonal disorders and sterility cases, it is useful in resolving suspicions of polycystic ovaries (see p 87), ovarian dysgenesis (see p 76), endometriosis (see p 71), and peritubal adhesions (Fig. 40).

An alternative procedure is culdoscopy, in which the cul-de-sac of Douglas is opened with a trocar, and a laparoscope is inserted to inspect the uterus and adnexa.

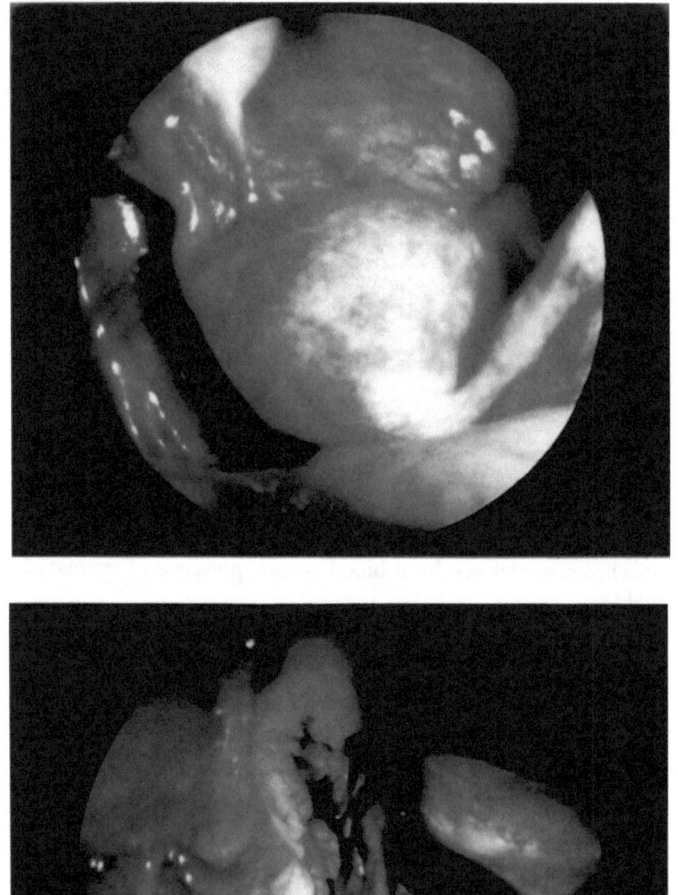

a

b

Fig. 39. a Normal laparoscopic photograph showing uterus, proximal portions of tubes and right ovary. **b** Laparoscopic photograph showing discharge of indigo carmine solution from the fimbriated end of a patent tube

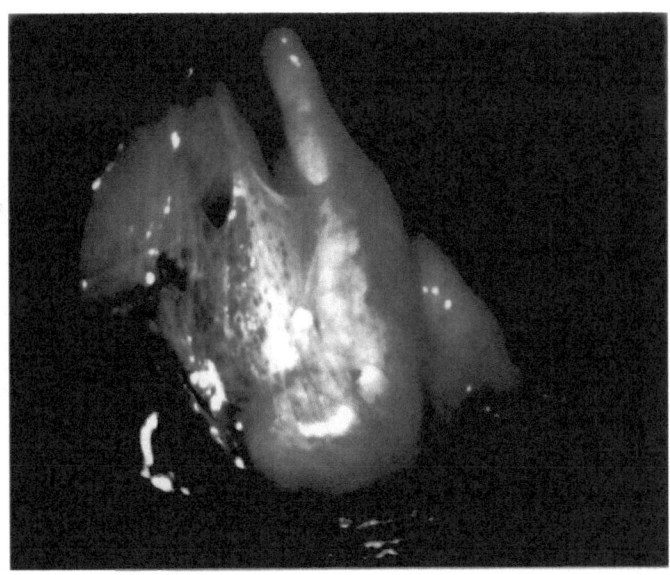

Fig. 40. Laparoscopic photograph showing tubal occlusion due to peritubal adhesions

7. Cranial X-Ray

Radiography of the sella turcica (Fig. 41 a, b) to exclude a pituitary tumor is always indicated in the presence of unexplained galactorrhea, cushingoid, or acromegalic symptoms, visual disturbances (particularly, narrowing of the visual field), and repeatedly high prolactin values in excess of 50 ng/ml.

In interpreting the pictures, it is important to remember that an adenoma of the anterior pituitary often does not cause noticeable distension of the sella turcica for some time. It is suggested, therefore, that a tomography is performed if the above symptoms are present.

8. Further Investigations

Since sterility is very often the first complaint associated with hormonal disorders in gynecology, it is important to touch upon the principal nonendocrinologic methods of diagnosis when infertility is present.

a) Semen Examination

When evaluating a couple for sterility, the physician should always assess the fertility of the male partner before investigating the hormonal status of the woman. For this purpose, following three days of abstinence, a semen specimen is

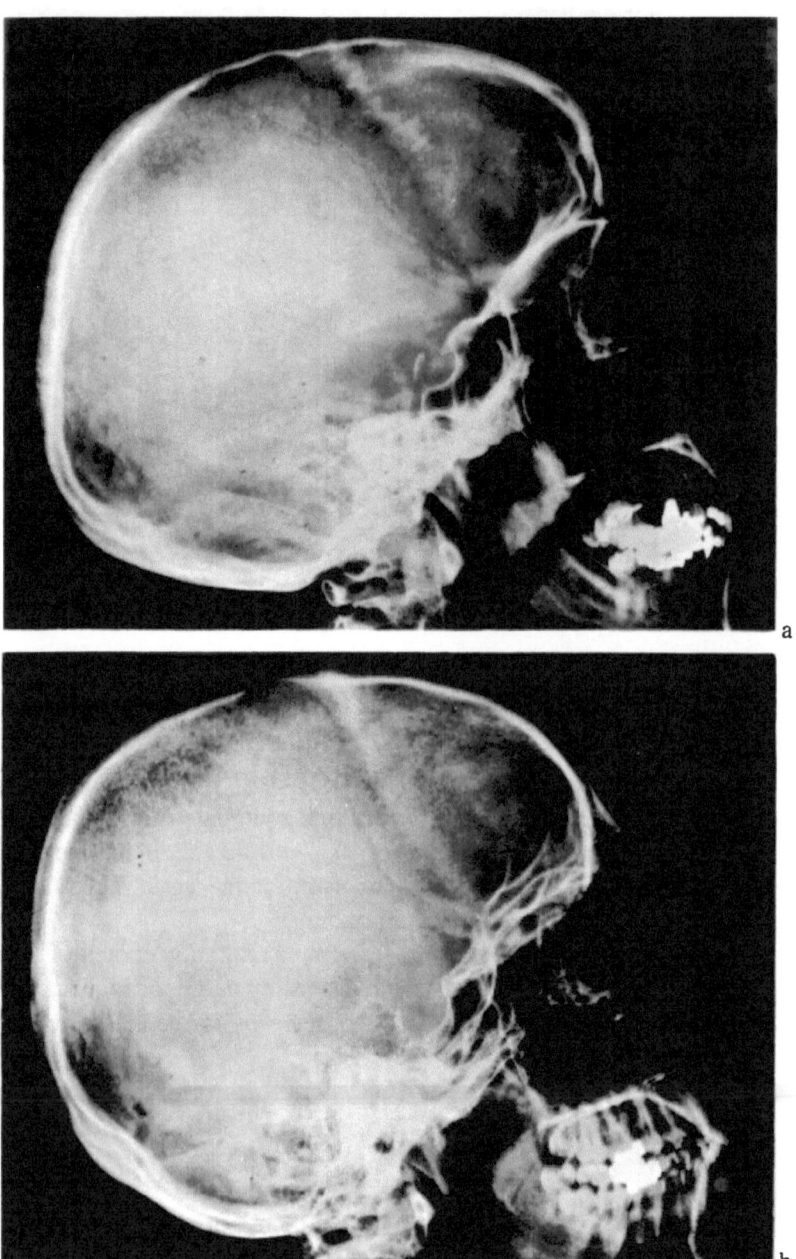

Fig. 41. a Normal sella turcica. b Distortion of sella turcica by prolactinoma of the pituitary

collected, by masturbation or by the use of a condom. The specimen should be examined within 2 h after collection. The study includes determination of the total volume, the number of sperm per ml, the percentage motility, and sperm morphology. Following the volume measurement, two portions of the specimen are taken up into leukocyte pipettes; one is diluted with methylene blue and the other with

38

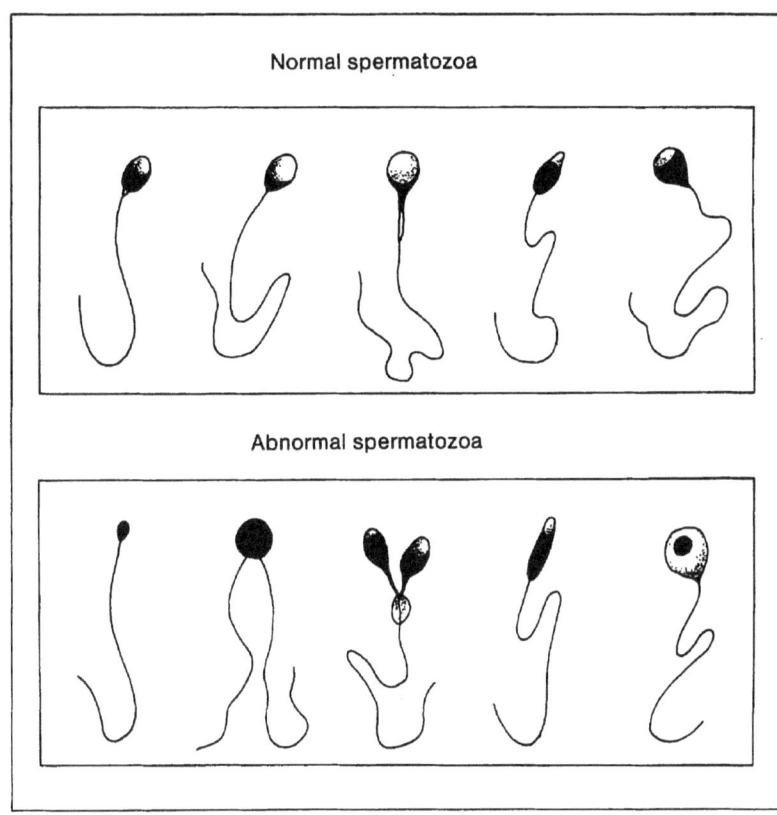

Fig. 42. Normal and abnormal spermatozoa

Table 3. Normal results of semen analysis

Quantity of ejaculate	2–8 ml
Sperm count	60–200 million
Motility	40–60%
2 h after ejaculation	
Differentiation	
Normal head shapes	80–90%
Abnormal head shapes	10–20%

physiologic saline, both in a ratio of 1:10 or 1:20. They are placed separately into a counting chamber; the first specimen is counted for the total number of spermatozoa, the second only for the number of dead sperm. The percentage of motile spermatozoa is calculated from the difference. For the evaluation of sperm morphology, which requires an experienced eye, a smear is prepared and stained with methylene blue or hematoxylin-eosin. The main types of normal and abnormal spermatozoa are illustrated in Fig. 42.

The values for normal semen are given in Table 3. It should be emphasized that unfavorable values do not necessarily denote sterility, for the range of subfertility is quite broad. Absolute infertility is indicated only by the complete absence of sperm, sperm counts below 1 million/ml, or a lack of motility. In any event, a second or even third specimen must be examined before a final appraisal is made.

b) Postcoital Test (Sims-Huhner Test)

Even with a normal semen analysis, an incompatibility may exist between the cervical mucus and the spermatozoa, which renders the sperm immotile. To exclude this immunologically determined sterility factor, a mucus specimen is taken from the cervical canal with a pipette or dissecting forceps 4–12 h following intercourse. The specimen is placed on a glass slide, topped by a coverslip, and immediately examined under high power magnification ($\sim$ 300 $\times$). Normally, at least five progressively motile sperm will be seen per high power field.

A positive result is obtained only under optimal mucus conditions, i. e., at midcycle (see p 28). Thus, the test is ordinarily performed between the 11th and 14th day of the cycle, at which time the cervical mucus should be clear with a *spinnbarkeit* of at least 4 cm. Also, the fern test (see p 32) should show good arborization, and only isolated leukocytes should be present. Of course the woman must refrain form douching or inserting chemical preparations into the vagina for at least 2 days prior to the test; sexual abstinence for a few days is also recommended.

Occasionally, neither motile nor immotile spermatozoa are found, despite good cervical mucus and a normal sperm analysis. This implies faulty sexual technique, rather than incompatibility, and tactful inquiry by the physician can help pinpoint the cause.

c) Tubal Insufflation

Tubal insufflation is a procedure which tests the patency of the fallopian tubes by the introduction of CO_2 into the uterus. The most favorable time is between cycle days 8 and 12, following the exclusion of inflammatory genital disease. The apparatus of Rubin or of Fikentscher and Semm, with or without a kymograph, has proved most serviceable.

Following a careful gynecologic examination, the patient is sedated with Valium or Spasmalgin. A vacuum-type cervical adapter with insufflation cannula is applied, and insufflation is begun at a flow rate of 30–120 ml/min. The pressure is increased every 30–60 s in increments of about 50 mm Hg to a maximum of 250 mm Hg. If occlusion is present, it can be lateralized by auscultation over each side of the lower abdomen. A tubal stenosis can also be localized by its characteristic sound during insufflation.

Normal tubes are patent at pressures of 40–100 mm Hg; if the device is equipped with a kymograph, a characteristic tracing is obtained (Fig. 43 a). Higher values indicate stenosis. If there is no passage of gas at a pressure of 200 mm Hg (Fig. 43 b), it probably signifies total occlusion of both tubes.

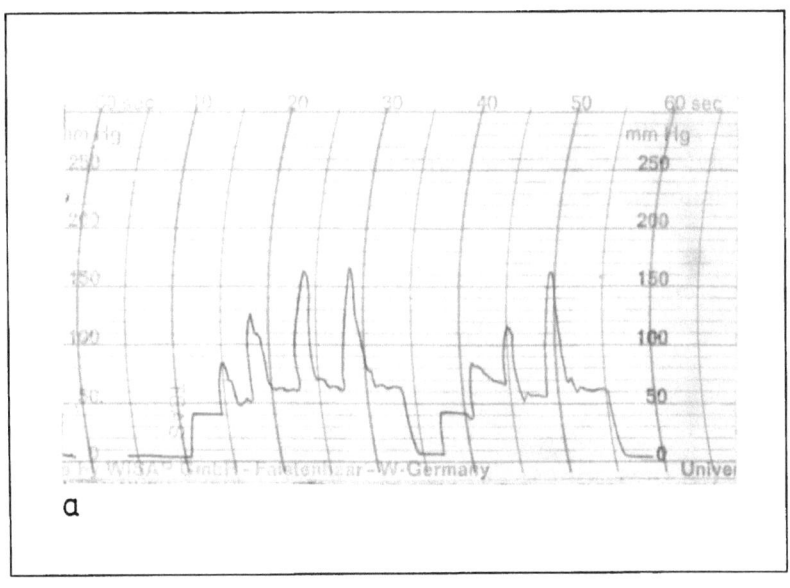

a

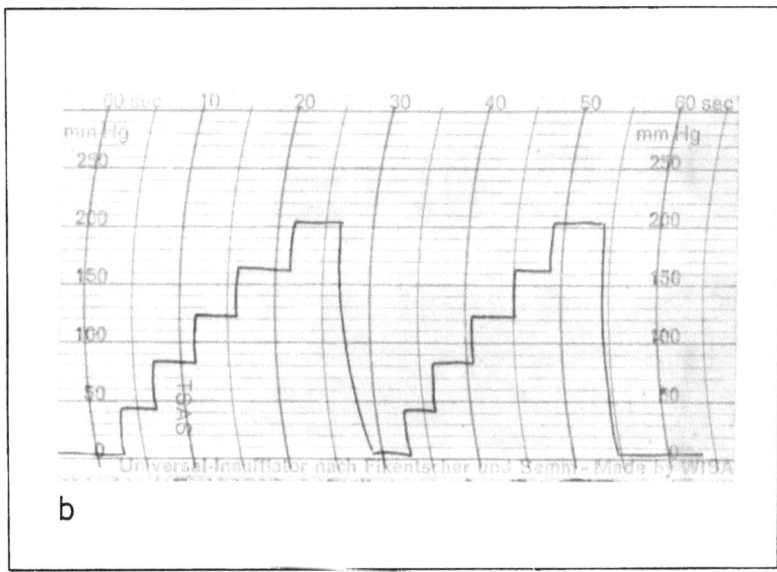

b

Fig. 43. a Kymographic trace showing normal tubal patency. **b** Trace showing bilateral tubal occlusion

In doubtful cases, confirmatory evidence of patency is afforded by the absence of hepatic dullness on percussion, the radiologic demonstration of a subphrenic gas shadow, and the patient's report of shoulder pain. A positive result is proof of patency but does not exclude peritubal adhesions or endometriosis. If the result is negative, the insufflation test must be repeated before a diagnosis of occlusion may be made.

d) Hysterosalpingography

The roentgenographic visualization of the uterus and tubes with a liquid contrast medium, e. g., Telebrix, is a more complicated procedure than insufflation and necessitates some degree of radiation exposure. By the same token, however, it yields more accurate information on the site of tubal stricture, while simultane-

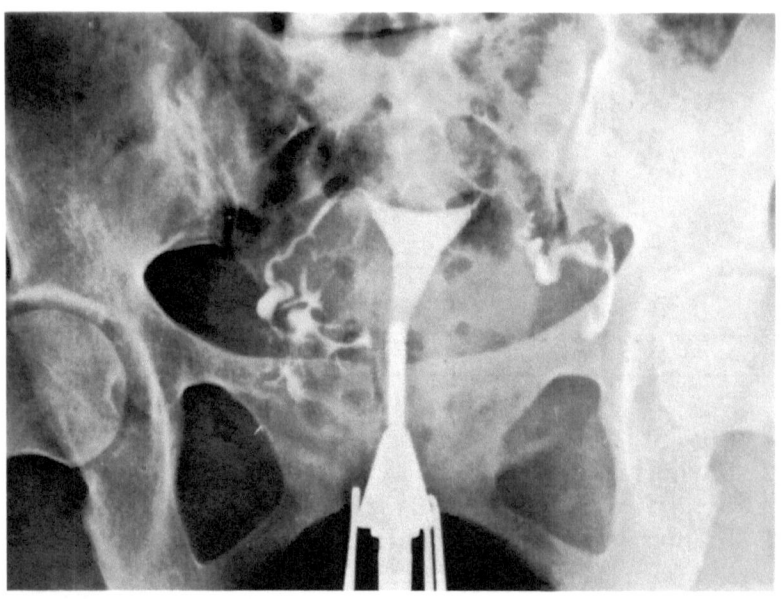

a

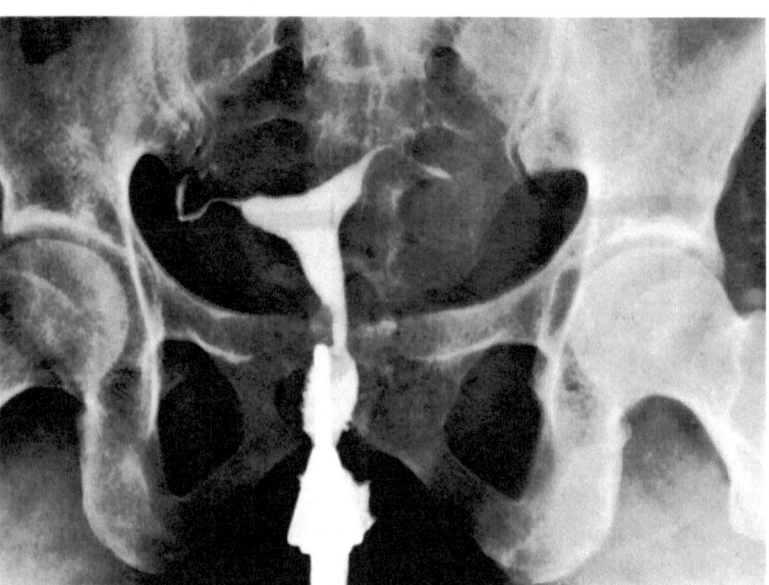

b

Fig. 44. a Normal hysterosalpingogram. **b** Hysterosalpingogram showing bilateral tubal occlusion

ously visualizing the interior of the uterus. Like all X-ray studies of the pelvic area, it is done only in the first half of the cycle to avoid possible irradiation of a fertilized ovum. Sterile precautions are of paramount importance. Latent infections are excluded by blood sedimentation, and prophylactic antibiotics are administered if necessary. The patient should be adequately sedated, but general anesthesia is rarely warranted. Following thorough vaginal disinfection, the lip of the cervix is mobilized with a tenaculum, and a uterine cannula or balloon catheter is introduced into the uterine cavity. From 2 to 8 ml of the contrast medium is injected. The first anteroposterior exposure of the pelvic cavity is taken immediately and a second after 1–2 min; more exposures may be taken at further intervals if desired (Fig. 44 a, b). An image amplifier can be used to trace the passage of the solution through the uterus and tubes. In unclear cases, a follow-up exposure taken several hours later is valuable in verifying release and distribution of the contrast medium in the peritoneal cavity.

IV. Hormone Assays

There are so many methods available at present for the determination of hormones that it is impossible to survey them all. We shall limit our discussion, therefore, to those methods of greatest practical importance, pointing out their usefulness as diagnostic tools. The specialized literature should be consulted for technical details.

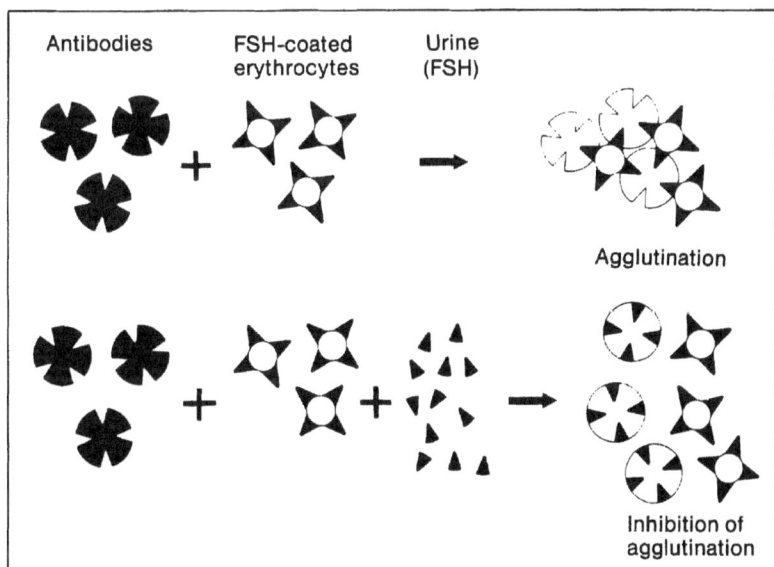

Fig. 45. Schema of the assay of FSH in the urine by hemagglutination inhibition. *Top,* no assayable FSH → agglutination of erythrocytes. *Bottom,* assayable FSH present → inhibition of hemagglutination

1. Pituitary Gonadotropins

The pituitary gonadotropins are of considerable importance in the diagnosis of endocrinologic diseases in gynecology. By determining the levels of FSH and LH, it is possible to classify patients into hypo-, normo-, and hypergonadotropic groups, which is of great prognostic and therapeutic value (see p 73). Low concentrations are indicative of severe hypothalamic-pituitary deficiency, while normal values are present in mild irregularities of gonadotropic secretion with no demonstrable ovarian or pituitary dysfunction. Elevated gonadotropins indicate ovarian failure, as encountered in postmenopause.

Today, FSH and LH may be determined by the hemagglutination inhibition method or, preferably, by radioimmunoassay. These methods have largely supplanted the bioassay of total gonadotropins by the mouse uterus test, of FSH by the augmentation test, and of LH by the ascorbic acid depletion test or the ventral prostatic weight test in infant rats.

Assay by hemagglutination inhibition corresponds essentially to a semiquantitative pregnancy test. It has been simplified by the availability of commercial reagent kits (FSH Nosticon, Luteonosticon, Organon) and can be performed even in non-

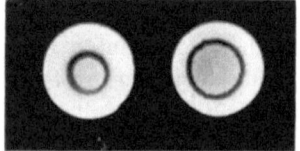 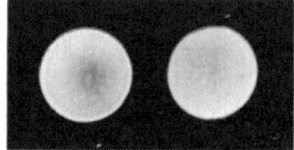

Fig. 46. Hemagglutination patterns in the assay of FSH and LH by hemagglutination inhibition. *Left*, positive result; *right*, negative result

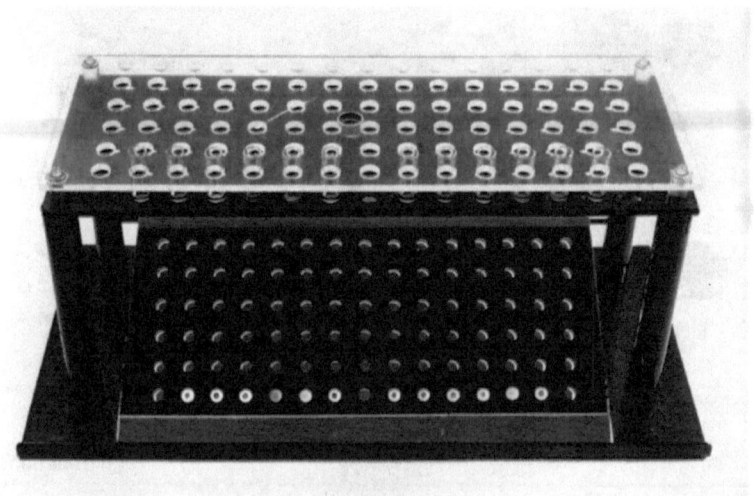

Fig. 47. Sedimentation rack for gonadotropin assay by hemagglutination inhibition, with tubes inserted

44

specialized laboratories. It is based on the competitive inhibition of the hemagglutination of FSH- or HCG-coated sheep erythrocytes by a specific antiserum in the presence of FSH or LH in the urine (Fig. 45). If sufficient quantities of the hormone are present in graded dilutions of the urine, the hormone binds to the antiserum, preventing it from agglutinating the antigen-coated erythrocytes. If on

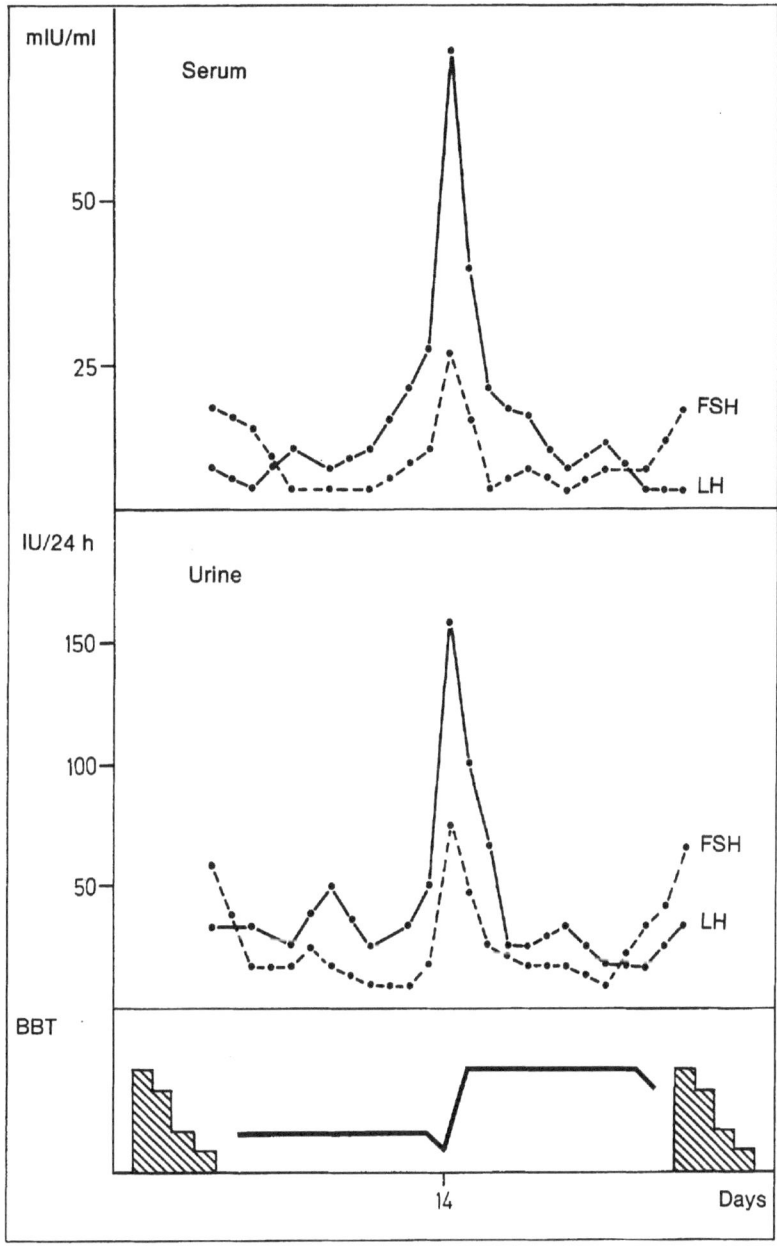

Fig. 48. FSH and LH levels in the serum and urine during a normal cycle as determined by radioimmunoassay and hemagglutination inhibition

the other hand, insufficient hormone is present, hemagglutination occurs. The reaction can be observed in special sedimentation tubes. The inhibition of agglutination is indicated by a reddish-brown ring, while agglutination leads to diffuse sedimentation (Figs. 46, 47).

Of course the results are not quantitative, but repeated assays are generally sufficient for the classification of cases and for simple endocrine diagnosis. Normal values during the reproductive years are 5–20 IU FSH and 20–100 IU LH, except at midcycle, when values may rise to 100 IU FSH and 600 IU LH per 24 h. After menopause, the FSH values range from 20 to 200, and the LH values from 100 to 600 IU per 24 h (Fig. 48 and Table 4). Since values are expressed in immunologic units, which cannot be compared with other results, the method must be specified.

The most reliable method for the determination of gonadotropins in the serum is radioimmunoassay, which requires special laboratory facilities. It is based on the competitive binding of the unknown hormone and a certain quantity of the same hormone radiolabeled with ^{125}I or ^{131}I to a highly specific antiserum (Fig. 49). A sample containing large quantities of hormone will occupy most of the binding sites on the antibodies, leaving few for the labeled hormone. The bound and unbound hormones are separated by chemical, physical, or immunologic means, and the radioactivity is counted in a gamma spectrometer (Fig. 50). The concentration of hormone in the sample is then calculated directly from a standard curve.

The method has been simplified considerably by commercial reagent kits (CIS, Amersham, Biolab, NEN), some of which are equipped with high-purity ^{125}I-labeled hormone in addition to the antiserum and buffer solutions. Experience with the method and a suitable spectrometer are still necessary, however.

Table 4. Normal values for pituitary gonadotropins

		Fertile women		Postmeno-pause
		Proliferative and secretory phase	Ovulatory	
Urine	FSH Hemagglutination inhibition	5–20 IU/24 h	10–100 IU/24 h	20–200 IU/24 h
	LH Hemagglutination inhibition	20–100 IU/24 h	150–600 IU/24 h	100–600
Serum	FSH (RIA)	2–20 mIU/ml	10–20 mIU/ml	20–200 mIU/ml
	LH (RIA)	2–20 mIU/ml	20–100 mIU/ml	20–100 mIU/ml

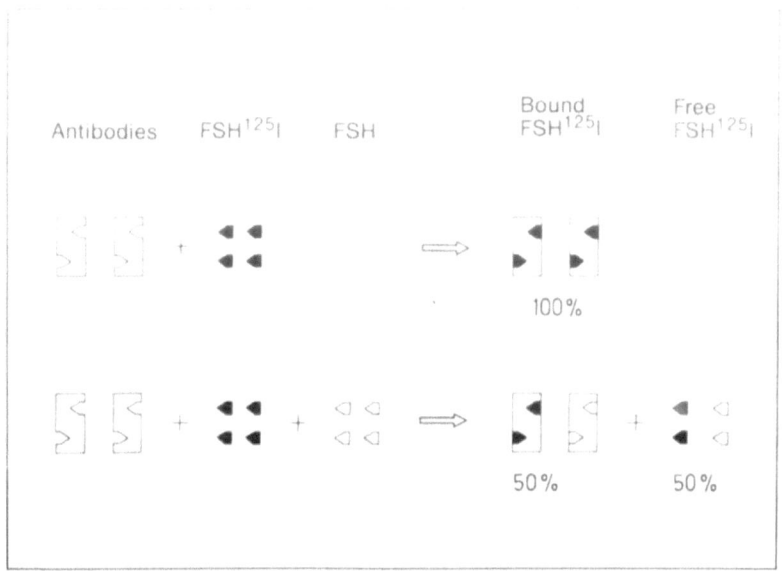

Fig. 49. Principle of the radioimmunoassay of FSH. *Top*, no assayable FSH → all FSH. →^{125}I bound. *Bottom*, assayable FSH present → FSH only partially ^{125}I bound

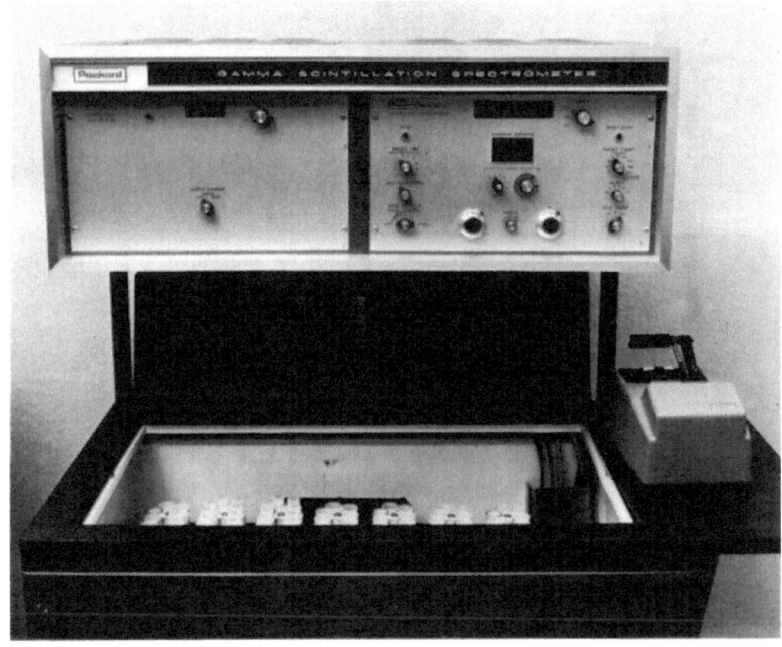

Fig. 50. Automatic gamma counter (Packard)

During childbearing years the normal values for FSH are 2–20 mIU/ml serum, and 2–100 mIU/ml for LH. After menopause the range is 20–200 mIU/ml serum (Fig. 48 and Table 4).

2. Prolactin

The determination of prolactin has aroused considerable interest in recent years. It is particularly indicated when galactorrhea is diagnosed in association with amenorrhea and other endocrine disorders (see p 85) and may be useful in other menstrual abnormalities and unexplained sterility.

The traditional bioassay methods have been abandoned in favor of radioimmunoassay, which yields very accurate results. Its principle is the same as in the determination of FSH and LH, and commercial reagent kits for prolactin are available (CIS).

The normal range is 6–20 ng/ml for all age groups. Mild hyperprolactinemia is seldom associated with demonstrable organic changes, but is rather due to the use of neuroleptics, oral contraceptives, and other drugs, or to emotional stress. Pituitary tumors can cause massive increases in prolactin, in which case values of 200–1000 ng/ml are not uncommon.

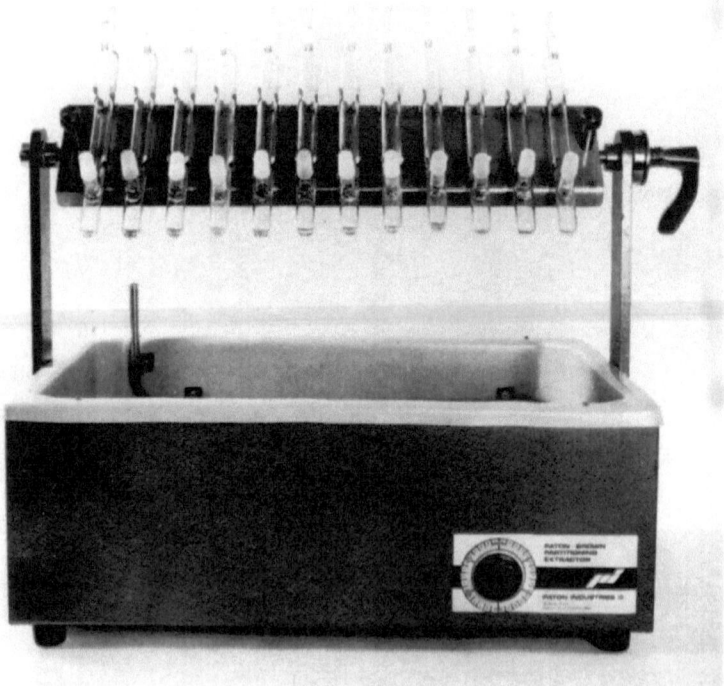

Fig. 51. Semiautomatic extractor for determining total urinary estrogens by the Brown method

3. Estrogens

Estrogen assays are of less practical importance than gonadotropin assays, because simple clinical methods such as vaginal cytology, cervical mucus examination, and the gestagen test afford good presumptive evidence of estrogen production. In more difficult cases, however, assays are indispensible for differential diagnosis

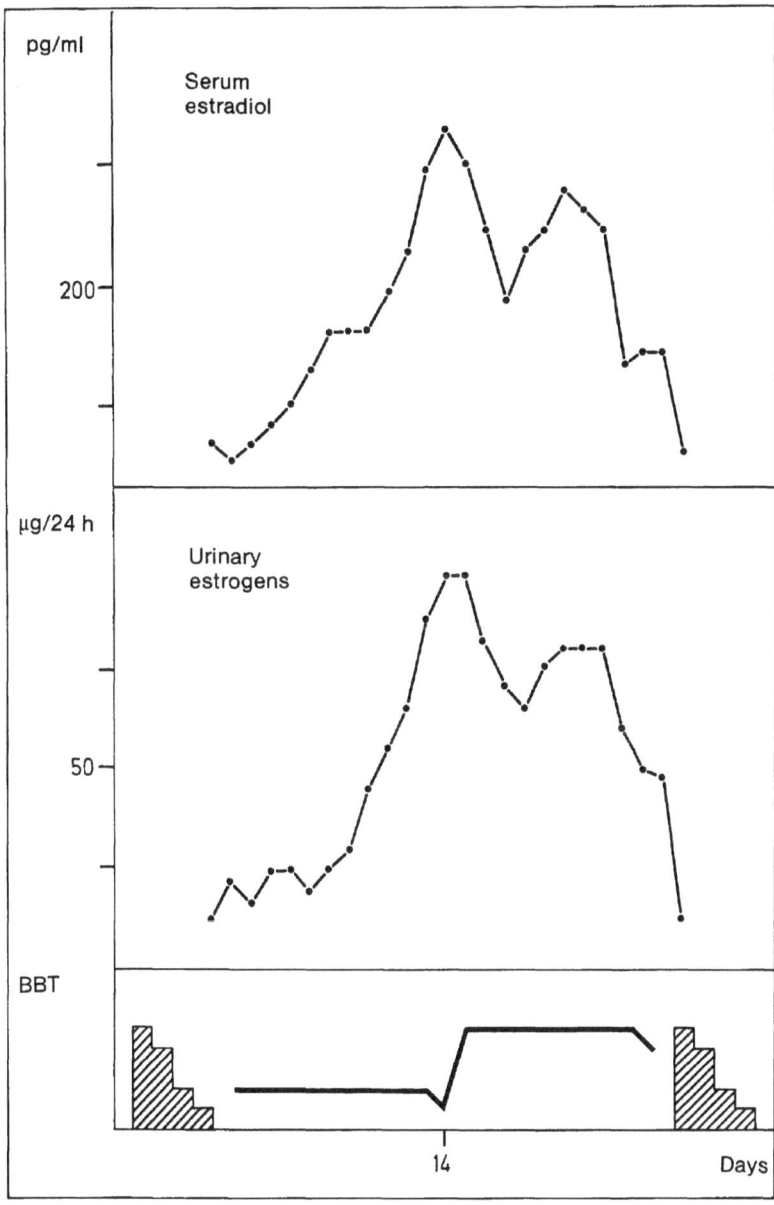

Fig. 52. Estrogen levels in the plasma and urine during a normal cycle as determined by radioimmunoassay and fluorometric assay, respectively

and for monitoring the results of treatment. The main indication for estrogen assay, aside from pregnancy, is in the diagnosis of hypoestrogenic, autonomic ovarian failure (see p 73), the detection of hormone-producing tumors (see p 94), and above all, the determination of the optimal time for ovulation induction with HCG following treatment with human gonadotropins (see p 84). A total estrogen assay is usually performed in the urine. The method of Brown, which uses a semiautomatic extractor (Fig. 51), has proved valuable for this purpose. Following acid hydrolysis, the estrogens are extracted and purified; then they are reacted with hydroquinone and sulfuric acid and measured fluorometrically after extraction with p-nitrophenol and tetrachlorethane. Fractionated assays of the three main urinary estrogens, estriol, estrone, and estradiol, are possible by means of column, thin-layer, or gas chromatography. The radioimmunoassay of serum estrogens, particularly estradiol-17 β, has attained considerable importance in recent years, and a number of corresponding reagent kits are available. In experienced hands, this technique has numerous advantages. However, for the time being it is restricted to centers which have the prerequisite equipment, especially a gamma or liquid scintillation counter.

Estrogen production during the reproductive years is strongly dependent on the menstrual cycle. In the proliferative phase, the excretion of total estrogens varies from 5 to 30 µg/24 h and the serum estradiol from 100 to 300 pg/ml. Peak values occur just before ovulation and can reach more than 100 µg/24 h and 600 pg/ml, respectively. A second, somewhat smaller peak usually occurs in the luteal phase (Fig. 52). After menopause the total estrogen excretion falls below 10 µg/24 h and the serum estradiol below 100 pg/ml (Table 5).

4. Progesterone and Pregnanediol

Progesterone and its excretory metabolite pregnanediol are determined mainly for the purpose of ovulation detection and assessement of luteal function. Where purely clinical questions are involved, the assays can often be dispensed with in favor of basal temperature charts (see p 20) and endometrial biopsy (see p 32).

Table 5. Normal estrogen values

		Fertile women			
		Proliferative phase	Ovula-tory	Luteal phase	Postmeno-pause
Urine	Total estrogens (flurorometric assay)	5–30 µg/24 h	50–150 µg/24 h	10–100 µg/24 h	2–10 µg/24 h
Serum	Estradiol (RIA)	100–300 pg/ml	300–600 pg/ml	100–300 pg/ml	10–50 pg/ml

Pregnanediol is best determined in a complete 24-h urine specimen. The method of Klopper has proved useful for this purpose; thin-layer chromatography has not proved satisfactory in all respects.

Depending on the method employed, pregnanediol excretion values of 0.5–2.5 mg/24 h are normal for the proliferative phase of the cycle and for anovulation; after ovulation the normal range is 4.5–7 mg/24 h (Fig. 53).

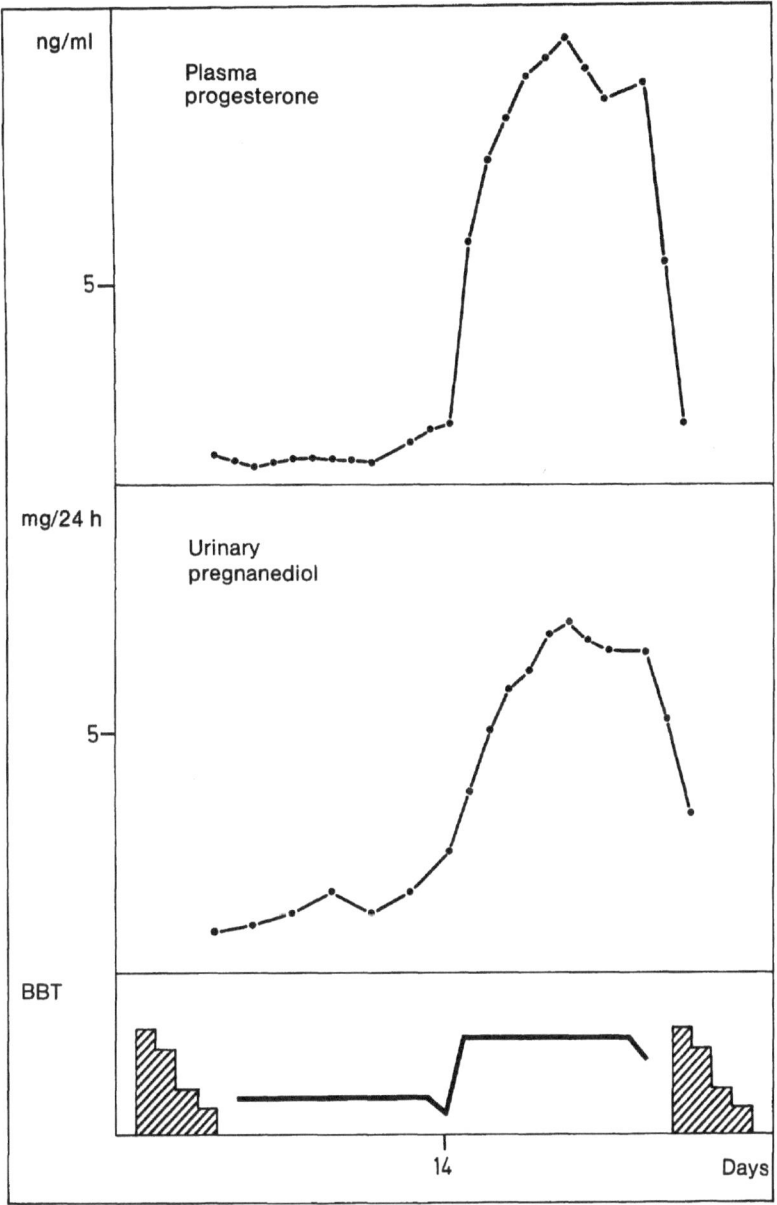

Fig. 53. Progesterone levels in the serum and pregnanediol excretion in the urine during a normal cycle as determined by radioimmunoassay and chemical assay, respectively

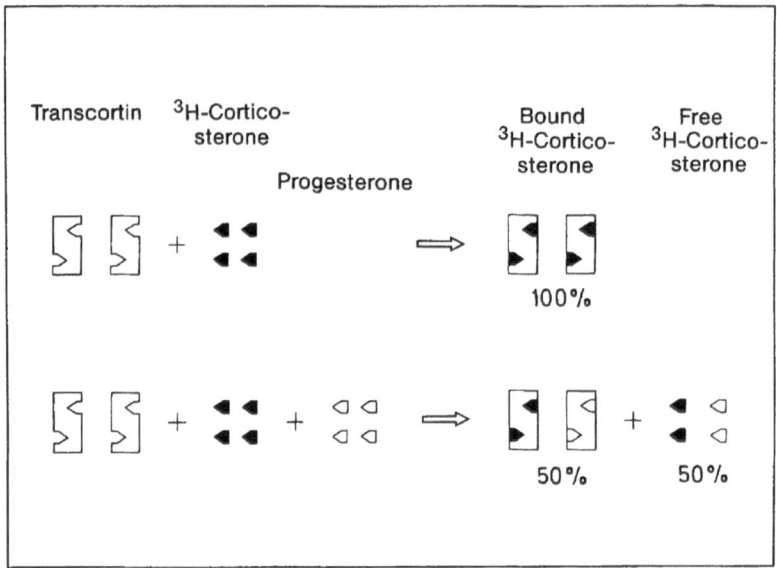

Fig. 54. Principle of progesterone assay by competitive protein binding. *Top,* no assayable progesterone → all ^{3}H-corticosterone bound. *Bottom,* assayable progesterone present → ^{3}H-corticosterone only partially bound

A more expedient method than determining the urinary metabolite is to measure the progesterone level in the serum. Again, the recommended technique is radioimmunoassay, employing the same procedure used for gonadotropins (see p 46) and other steroid hormones. Suitable reagent kits (CIS, Biolab) are available. Protein binding methods based on the competitive binding of progesterone and labeled corticosterone to transcortin (Fig. 54) have become somewhat less important by comparison. The normal values for serum progesterone in the proliferative phase are less than 1 ng/ml; the luteal peak on the 6th–10th day after ovulation is 10–30 ng/ml (Fig. 53).

5. 17-Ketosteroids and Testosterone

The determination of androgenic metabolites in gynecology is of considerably greater importance than might first be assumed. A common complaint among women today is hirsutism. It can be extremely difficult to differentiate clinically between "constitutional" hirsutism and the much rarer types of ovarian or adrenal origin, particularly if signs of true virilization, such as increased musculature, deepening of the voice, and clitoral hypertrophy are absent.

In all these cases the simplest screening method is the determination of urinary 17-ketosteroids, the principal degradation products of androgens from the adrenal cortex and ovary. The most important are androsterone, etiocholanolone, and dehydroepiandrosterone. Numerous assay methods have been developed for these

Table 6. Normal values for 17-ketosteroids and testosterone in females

Urine	17-Ketosteroids (chemical assay)	5–15 mg/24 h
Serum	Testosterone (RIA)	0.1–0.8 ng/ml

hormones. One of the most suitable for clinical purposes is the method of Peterson and Pierce, which consists of acid hydrolysis, extraction with petroleum ether and benzene, and a color reaction with *m*-dinitrobenzene (Zimmerman reaction). The hormone concentration is measured spectrophotometrically, using dehydroepiandrosterone as the standard. The procedure is simple and can be done in any clinical laboratory.

Normal values for urinary 17-ketosteroids in women are 5–15 mg/24 h. There is a slight physiologic decline after menopause (Table 6). Elevations are found in adrenocortical hyperplasia, androgen-producing ovarian tumors, testicular feminization (see p 77), and occasionally in the Stein-Leventhal syndrome (see p 87). Tumors of the adrenal cortex are associated with a substantial increase. If elevated values are found, further tests are warranted (see p 58ff.).

Fractionation of the 17-ketosteroids has been attempted as an aid to differential diagnosis. Indeed, a relative increase in the androsterone and etiocholanolone fractions is occasionally associated with ovarian tumors. However, reliable results are not obtained as a general rule.

The determination of plasma testosterone to evaluate hirsutism and exclude androgen-producing tumors is a more technically complex procedure but is superior in many respects to 17-ketosteroid assay. Today, radioimmunoassay methods are employed almost exclusively for routine purposes (see p 46). The testosterone values in normal women are 0.1–0.8 ng/ml. Values in excess of 10 ng/ml may occur in virilzing diseases; elevations also occur during pregnancy. Lately, the determination of other androgen metabolites, such as serum androstenedione and dehydroepiandrosterone, has gained increasing differential diagnostic importance.

6. 17-Hydroxycorticoids, Cortisol, Corticosterone

The identification of corticosteroids and their degradation products plays a more or less supplementary role in gynecologic endocrinology, although it has become promising as a more defintive diagnostic technique.

Urinary corticosteroids are usually determined in the form of 17-hydroxycorticoids, also called Porter-Silber chromogens. These are mainly the metabolites of cortisol and cortexolone, but not of corticosterone. They can be analyzed simply by the method of Petersen, which requires enzymatic hydrolysis with β-glucuronidase, extraction with methylene chloride, and treatment with phenylhydrazine indicator, followed by spectrophotometric assay. An alternate method is to determine the urinary 17-ketogenic steroids; the cortisol metabolites, as well as pregnanetriol, are measured by this technique.

Plasma corticosteroid assays are preferred for many applications, particularly function tests (see p 58). The most suitable techniques are fluorometry and radioimmunoassay. A specific cortisol assay is possible, but often corticosterone is determined along with the much more abundant cortisol in routine studies.

The normal patient has a urinary excretion of 3–12 mg/24 h for 17-hydroxycorticosteroids, and 5–16 mg/24 h for 17-ketogenic steroids. The normal values for plasma cortisol range from 5 to 25 µg/100 ml and show a diurnal variation. Levels are elevated in Cushing's syndrome and reduced in Addison's disease and panhypopituitarism.

7. Thyroxin

When clinical features suggest hypo- or hyperfunction of the thyroid gland, the simplest confirmatory test is the determination of serum thyroxine, or T_4, by radioimmunoassay. In contrast to the traditional but now obsolete protein-bound iodine (PBI) test, radioimmunoassay is specific and is unaffected by iodides or organic dyes.

The normal range is 4–11 µg/100 ml. Results can be falsely elevated during pregnancy, by the use of estrogens or oral contraceptives, and in hepatitis. Spurious reductions are occasionally caused by renal disease as well as by salicylates and diphenylhydantoin. On the whole, these readings reflect a shift of specific binding proteins in the serum, which can be quickly recognized by use of the triiodothyronine (T_3) uptake test.

The further evaluation of a diagnosed thyroid disease, which must include radioiodine studies and accurate tests of central regulation, is best left to the specialized endocrinologist.

V. Function Tests

The purpose of function tests is to test the response of an endocrine system to hormones or hormone antagonists. The diagnostic value of such a dynamic test is superior to that of purely static methods, although correspondingly greater effort and expense are generally required.

1. Gestagen Test

The gestagen test (progesterone test) is the most important and most informative function test for the evaluation and classification of patients with amenorrhea. It can be performed on any patient and under any circumstances and involves the administration of relatively large doses of a synthetic gestagen. If the endometrium is properly estrogen-primed, uterine bleeding will ensue 2–4 days after the hormone is withdrawn or its effect subsides. For practical reasons the test is best performed with an orally active gestagen with no estrogenic activity, such as 10 mg Orgametril (Organon) or 20 mg Primolut N (Schering), daily for 6 days (Fig. 55). A positive result, i. e., the occurrence of withdrawal bleeding, indicates adequate ovarian estrogen production and a responsive endometrium. A negative result indicates estrogen deficiency secondary to autonomic ovarian failure, an absent or unresponsive endometrium, or early pregnancy, in which case withdrawal bleeding is prevented by endogenous estrogen and progesterone production.

2. Estrogen Test

If the gestagen test is negative, the estrogen test may be done to aid in further differentiation. In this test estrogens are administered over a number of days to stimulate endometrial proliferation. Normally, discontinuance of the hormone will evoke withdrawal bleeding. Orally active synthetic estrogens are recommended, such as 0.1 mg Lynoral (Organon) or Progynon C (Schering) daily for 2 weeks (Fig. 56). A positive result verifies the presence of a responsive endometrium, while a negative result indicates amenorrhea of uterine origin, except during pregnancy.

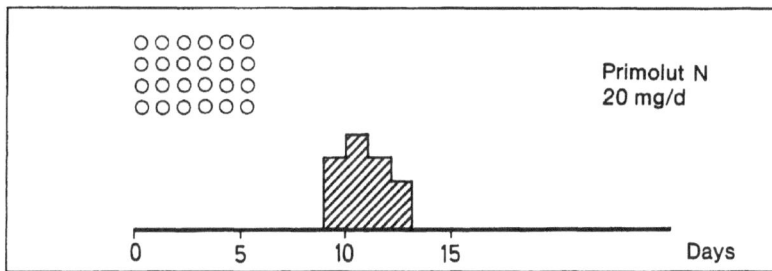

Fig. 55. Schema of the gestagen test

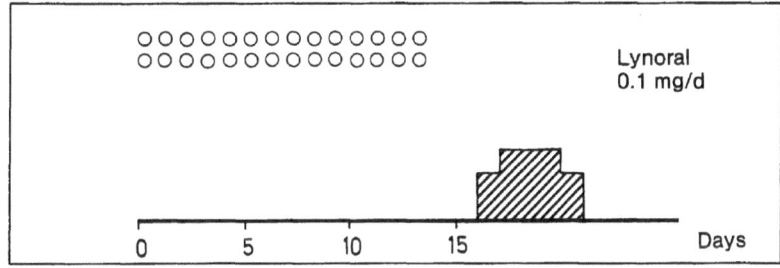

Fig. 56. Schema of estrogen test

3. Gonadotropin Test

Gonadotropins can also be administered as a direct test of ovarian responsiveness in the event of a negative gestagen test due to autonomic ovarian failure. The test is reliable only if costly human gonadotropins are used, such as Pergonal (Serono) or Humegon (Organon). Following prolonged stimulation, estrogen production is directly assessed or estimated indirectly by changes in the vaginal smear and cervical mucus (see p 28). A positive result indicates an intact germinal parenchyma; a negative result after adequate dosing is indicative of ovarian failure. The test is of minimal importance, however, since the same differentiation can be accomplished more simply by gonadotropin assay (see p 44).

4. Clomiphene Test

The synthetic stilbene derivative clomiphene (Clomid, Merrell) can be administered to test hypothalamic function. Generally, this agent is used therapeutically rather than diagnostically as a means of inducing ovulation (see p 83). It blocks the estrogen receptors of the diencephalon, thereby causing a compensatory increase in the secretion of FSH and LH. In the function test, clomiphene is administered in a dose of 100–150 mg/day for 5 days. Before, during, and several days after this regime, the levels of FSH and LH are measured by radioimmunoassay (Fig. 57). Normally, both gonadotropins will rise to several times their initial levels. Positive results indicate good hypothalamic function and imply a favorable prognosis for

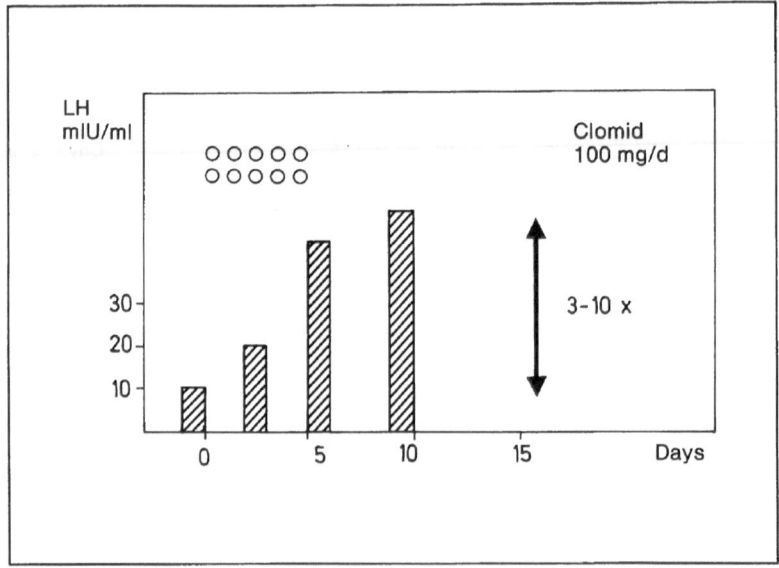

Fig. 57. Schema of the clomiphene test

treatment with centrally acting ovulation-inducing agents. Negative results are indicative of severe hypothalamic or pituitary dysfunction.

The test is complicated, costly, and therefore of limited practical importance. Moreover, it affords little more than the trial use of clomiphene with a purely clinical assessment.

5. Luteinizing Hormone Releasing Hormone Test

The responsiveness of the anterior pituitary can be tested directly by the adminis-tration of LH-releasing hormone (LH-RH). In some cases this test enables an accurate localization of the endocrine disorder and thus permits a specific therapy. Generally, 25–100 µg synthetic LH-RH is administered intravenously or intramuscularly. The serum LH is measured by radioimmunoassay (see p 46) before the injection, as well as 15, 30, 60, and 120 min afterward. If gonadotropin secretion by the anterior pituitary is normally responsive to RH, the injection will evoke a rapid, marked rise of the serum LH. If the pituitary is unresponsive, no rise will occur (Fig. 58a, b). Centrally acting agents such as Clomid and Fertodur (see p 82) are useful therapeutically only in patients with a positive LH-RH test. If the test is negative, gonadotropin replacement with Pergonal or Humegon (see p 84) is usually required.

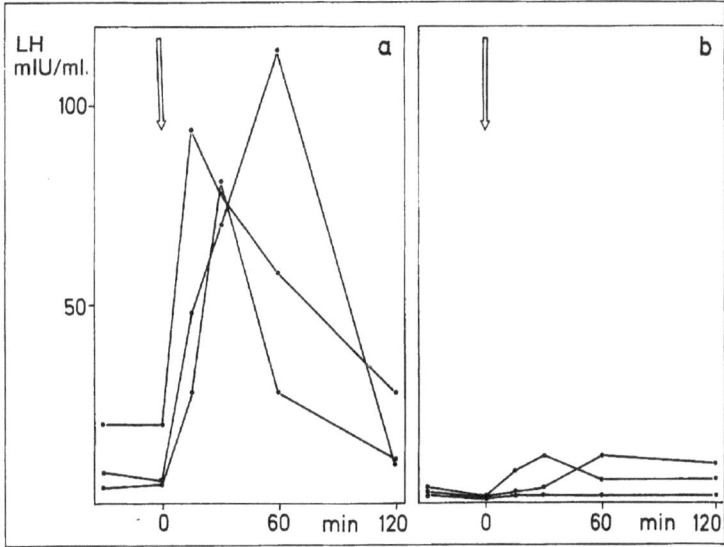

Fig. 58 a, b. LH-RH test with 25 µg LH-RH iv. **a** Good pituitary response. **b** No pituitary response

6. Adrenocorticotrophic Hormone Test

Adrenocorticotrophic hormone (ACTH) loading is one of the most important tests of adrenal cortical function but is also useful in solving endocrinologic problems in gynecology. Several variants of this test are known. On an outpatient basis, the short test with synthetic ACTH such as Synacthen (Ciba) is recommended. A dose of 0.25 mg is administered intramuscularly in the morning; blood samples for

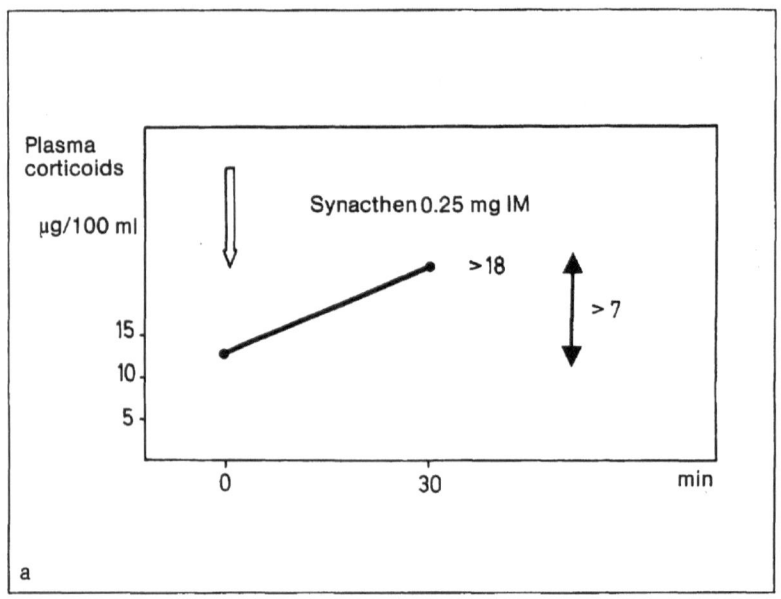

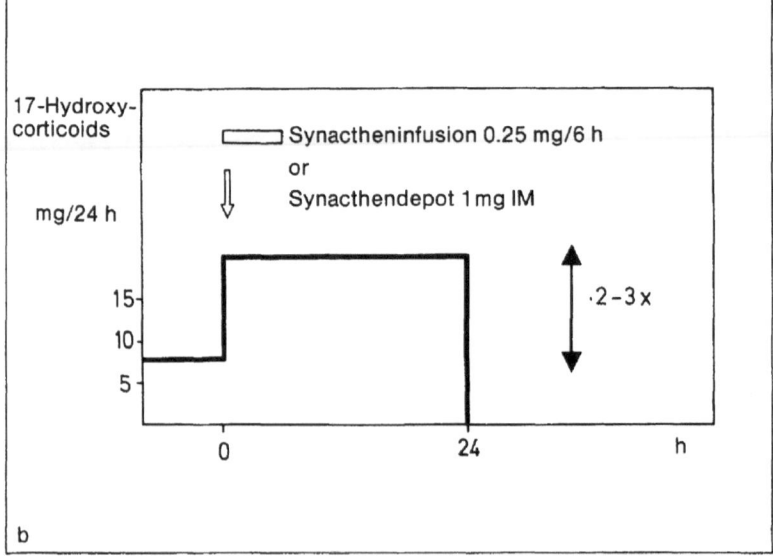

Fig. 59a, b. ACTH test with Synacthen. **a** Short test. **b** Standard test

plasma corticosteroid assay are taken immediately before and 30 min after the injection (Fig. 59a). Patients with normal adrenal cortical function show a rise of at least 7 µg/100 ml to a level exceeding 18 µg/100 ml. A smaller elevation is evidence of adrenal cortical insufficiency, while a greater rise indicates hyperplasia, as in Cushing's syndrome. Patients with functioning adrenocortical tumors show varying responses and may fail to show any rise, because the secretion is largely independent of the anterior pituitary. The longer, standard test requires hospitalization. In this test, ACTH is administered by infusion, e. g., 0.25 mg Synacthen for 6 h, or intramuscularly in a dose of 1 mg (Fig. 59b). Normally, the urinary excretion of 17-hydroxycorticoids should increase by a factor of 2–3 compared to the control urine collected earlier. This test may be ordered if results from the short test are equivocal.

The older test based on the induction of eosinopenia by the administration of ACTH has become largely obsolete.

7. Dexamethasone Suppression Test

This is perhaps the most important test of adrenal cortical function and measures the suppression of corticoid secretion following the administration of a potent glucocorticoid such as dexamethasone.

A short test has also been developed which makes a suitable office screening procedure: A blood sample is drawn at 8 A. M. for plasma corticoid assay (see p 54). The patient receives 1 mg of dexamethasone orally at midnight of the same day, and a second blood sample is drawn the next morning at 8 o'clock (Fig. 60a). In the normal patient the corticoid level falls by more than 50% to below 10 µg/100 ml. A smaller fall is indicative of Cushing's syndrome due to an adrenocortical or pituitary tumor. More accurate results can be obtained by administering dexamethasone for a period of several days. The patient is put on continuous 24-h urine collections for assay of 17-hydroxycorticoids and 17-ketosteroids for the duration of the test, and for the next 2 days receives 0.5 mg dexamethasone orally every 6 h (Fig. 60b). The normal patient will show a suppression of both steroid fractions by 50% or more of initial values to less than 4 mg/24 h; this is also the case in congenital adrenogenital syndrome. A smaller suppression is pathognomonic of Cushing's syndrome.

8. Metopirone Test

This third test of adrenal cortical function is somewhat less important than the two function tests previously described. Metopirone (Ciba) is an adrenocorticostatic which blocks 11-β-hydroxylation, thereby inhibiting the biosynthesis of cortisol and corticosterone. This causes a compensatory increase in ACTH secretion, which in normal individuals leads to an increased adrenal output of cortexolone

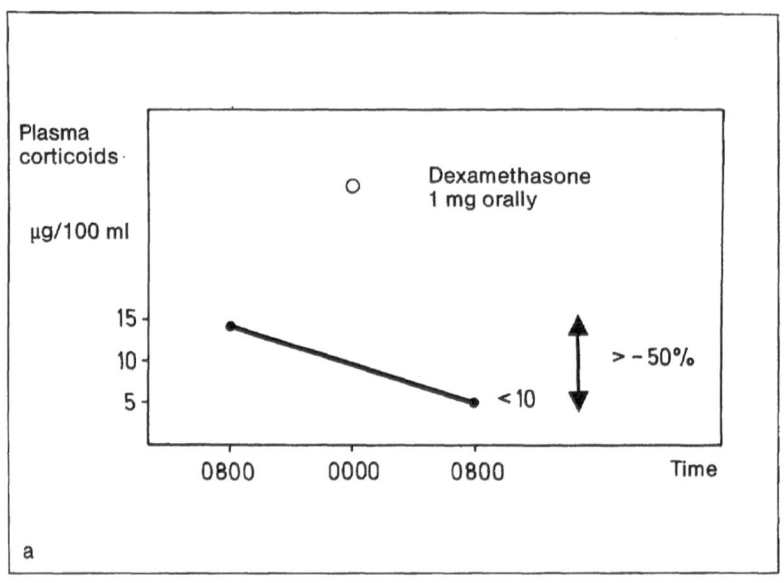

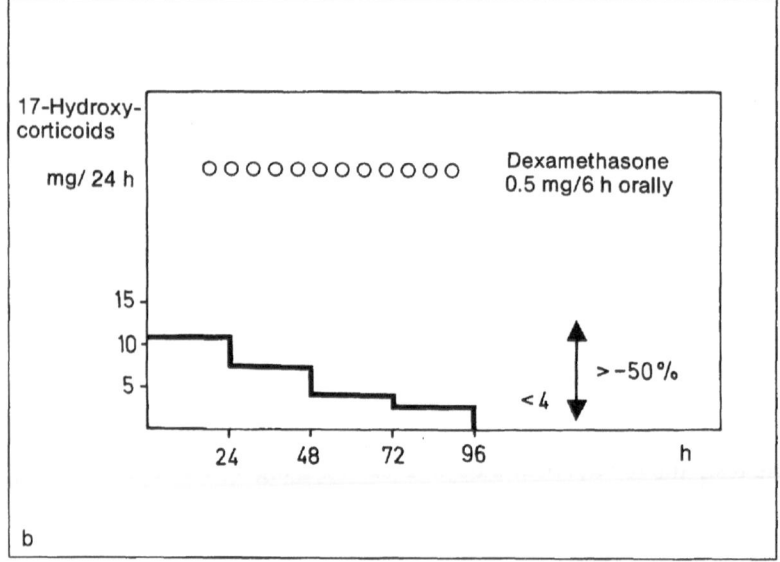

Fig. 60 a, b. Dexamethasone test. **a** Short test. **b** Standard test

(compound S) instead of cortisol. This results in a rise of urinary 17-hydroxycorticoids and 17-ketosteroids under normal circumstances.

This function test is best conducted on an inpatient basis. It is diagnostic only if positive. A 24-h urine sample is obtained on the first day to determine baseline values, then for the next 2 days 0.5 g Metopirone is administered orally every 4 h (Fig. 61). Continuous 24-h urine collections are made during this period and on the day following the last administration of Metopirone. In patients with normal pituitary and adrenocortical function, the urinary 17-hydroxycorticoids increase

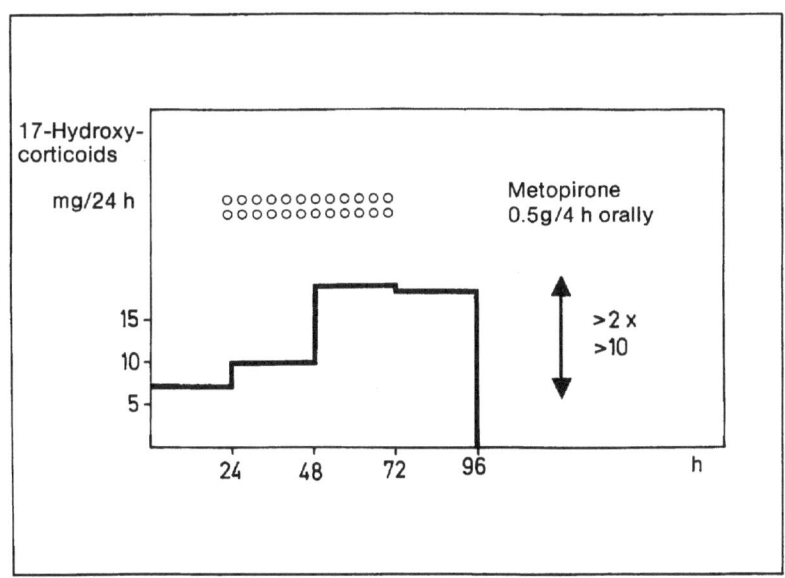

Fig. 61. Metopirone test

by at least a factor of 2, or by more than 10 mg/24 h, on the 3rd and 4th days of the test. A lack of response indicates a disturbance of ACTH secretion, as encountered in panhypopituitarism, pituitary tumors, and after prolonged cortisone therapy. The same results are obtained in cases of adrenocortical insufficiency and adrenocortical tumors, but these conditions also produce a negative ACTH test.

9. Dexamethasone-Human Chorionic Gonadotropin Test

This very special study has attained some importance in gynecology as a means of differentiating between an adrenal and ovarian cause of excessive androgen production. The patient is given 3 mg dexamethasone daily for 12 days. On the 6th, 7th, and 8th days an additional 5000 IU/day HCG (Pregnyl, Organon; Primogonyl, Schering) is administered intramuscularly (Fig. 62). The urinary 17-ketosteroids are repeatedly determined throughout the course of the test. In normal patients and patients with adrenal cortical hyperplasia, the values fall below 2 mg/24 h during dexamethasone administration and do not recover during administration of HCG. In patients with excessive ovarian androgen production (e. g., Stein-Leventhal syndrome), the fall of 17-ketosteroids is significantly smaller, and stimulation with HCG produces a substantial rise. The actual diagnostic value of this very costly and time-consuming test is a matter of dispute, however.

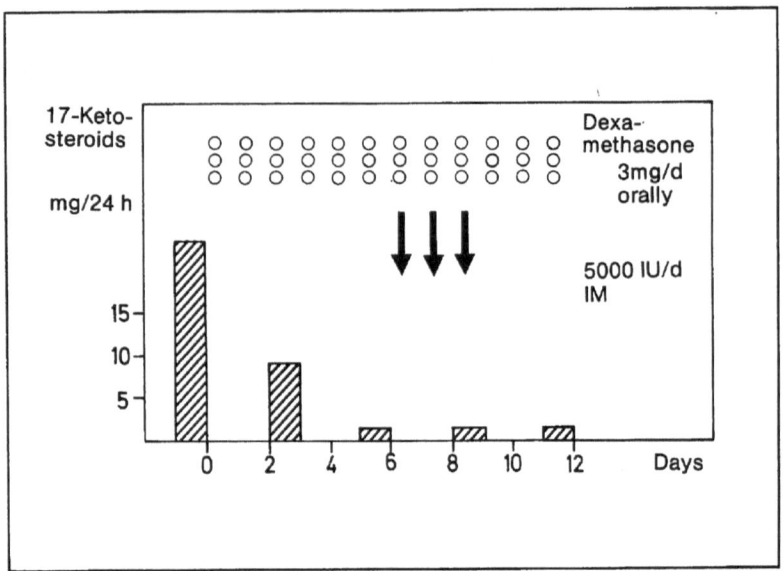

Fig. 62. Dexamethasone-HCG test

C. Important Hormonal Disorders in Gynecology

I. Menstrual Disorders

1. Abnormalities of Rhythm

Abnormalities in the rhythm of the menstrual cycle include infrequent menstruation, or oligomenorrhea, as well as menstruation at abnormally frequent intervals, or polymenorrhea (Fig. 63).

There are certain vagaries in the exact definition of these abnormalities. However, since 95% of menstrual cycles are from 21 to 35 days in duration during reproductive life, we may take this range as the "normal" periodicity and assume that only marked deviations constitute true abnormalities of rhythm.

a) Oligomenorrhea

The often scanty menstrual flows occur at intervals of 36–90 days. Longer menstrual intervals are considered to fall within the amenorrheal range (see p 73).

Pathogenesis. Oligomenorrhea may be primary, and thus in evidence since the menarche, or may arise secondarily during the reproductive years. It is usually the result of a hypothalamic dysfunction which, as in amenorrhea, is very often based upon emotional conflicts related to job, family, sexual activity, or a change of environment. Oligomenorrhea also occurs in other endocrine syndromes, such as disorders of the adrenal cortex and thyroid, as well as in obesity and anorexia. Polycycstic ovaries are also a common cause of this abnormality. Usually the cycles are anovulatory, although occasionally ovulation occurs after an extended proliferative phase.

Diagnosis. Besides the psychologic history and physical examination, it is important to obtain an accurate record of bleeding and basal temperature graph. Specific assays for hormones such as gonadotropins and estrogens and simple function studies such as the gestagen test are seldom very informative, since the results generally are in the mid- to low-normal range. On the other hand, prolactin assay, adrenocortical function tests, and the exclusion of thyroid disease can be helpful in certain cases.

Treatment. The therapy of choice, especially in younger patients, is to regulate the cycle with weak progestins such as Retroid (Roche) or Duphaston (Philips-Duphar) taken orally in daily doses of 4–12 mg for 10 days (Fig. 73, p 81). A portion of the patients will achieve regular menstruation after a few months' therapy, while others will require a longer course of treatment. About 20% may even achieve ovulation owing to the hypothalamic-stimulating effect of the medication. An acceptable alternative is Cyclacur (Schering), a weak estrogen-gestagen preparation which contains the natural estrogen estradiol valerate instead of artificial estrogens and thus causes no central inhibition. Oral contraceptives are strictly contraindicated, for they further suppress the already deficient hypothalamic control. In women who desire pregnancy, pharmacologic ovulation induction with Fertodur (Schering) or Clomid (Merrell) (see p 82) is indicated. Psychological guidance is an important adjunct, and a reducing diet should be prescribed for obese patients.

b) Polymenorrhea

This term is applied to menstrual bleeding that occurs at intervals of less than 21 days (Fig. 63).

Pathogenesis. The bleeding of polymenorrhea may be of the anovulatory withdrawal type or may be ovulatory with an abnormally short proliferative or secretory phase. Generally, the cause lies in a defect of hypothalamic control. Polymenorrhea is most common during the transitional phases of life, i. e., puberty and the climacteric.
A short luteal phase is of particular clinical importance. If it is shorter than 10 days in an ovulatory cycle, functional sterility will result. There are two variants of this defect according to etiology: a centrally determined, hypoluteotropic form with inadequate LH stimulation of the corpus luteum, and a hyperluteotropic form with defective steroid biosynthesis in the corpus luteum. In each case there is deficient secretory preparation of the endometrium and inadequate progesterone production during the second half of the cycle. As a result of this, the fertilized ovum is unable to implant.

Diagnosis. Polymenorrhea requires no special diagnostic tests, but an evaluation of luteal function is indicated in sterile patients. This can be done by means of the basal temperature graph (see p 20), endometrial biopsy, (see p 32) and the determination of progesterone or pregnanediol (see p 50).

Treatment. Polymenorrhea can be treated by the cyclic administration of an estrogen-gestagen preparation such as Cyclacur (Schering), Progylut (Schering), or oral contraceptives. Generally, though, treatment becomes necessary only if sterility is present. Anovulation is treated with Clomid (Merrell) or with Fertodur (Schering) (see p 82).

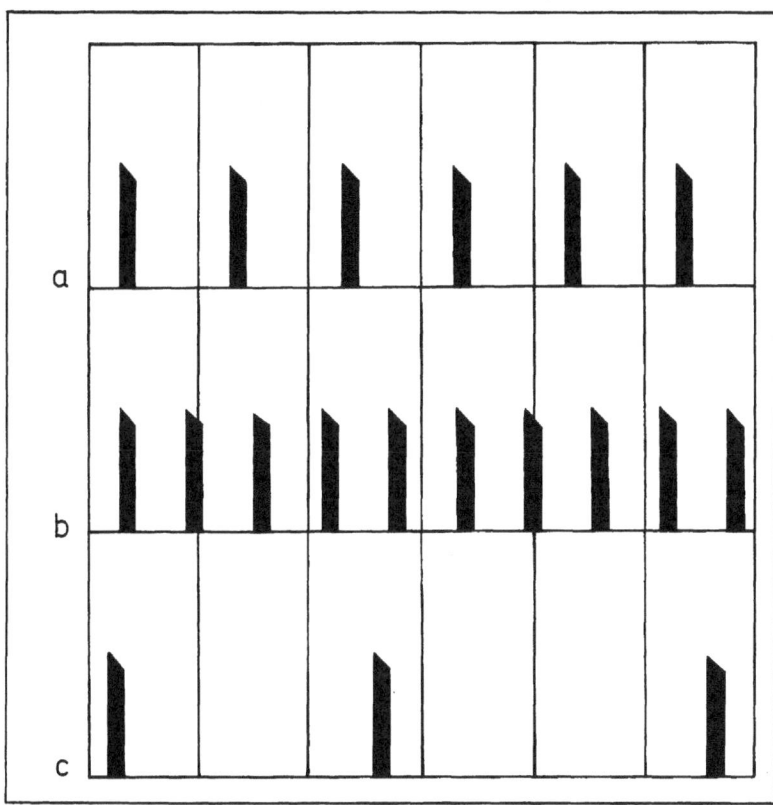

Fig. 63 a–c. Abnormalities of rhythm. **a** Eumenorrhea. **b** Polymenorrhea. **c** Oligomenorrhea

Biphasic cycles in which only the proliferative phase is shortened do not ordinarily require treatment, although ovulation can be delayed by administering, for example, 0.1 mg ethinyl estradiol (Lynoral, Organon; Progynon, Schering) daily from cycle day 3 through 10. Luteal inadequacy with a short luteal phase can be managed by replacement therapy with gestagens or estrogens, such as 25 mg progesterone intravaginally, or three tablets Primosiston (Schering) orally, daily for 10 days immediately after the midcycle thermal shift. An alternative is stimulation with chorionic gonadotropin. The recommended course is 1500–2500 IU HCG (Pregnyl, Organon; Primogonyl, Schering; Profasi, Serono) administered by intramuscular injection on the 4th, 7th, and 10th days after the rise of basal temperature; this produces a hyperthermal plateau of at least 12 days' duration as well as normal progesterone and pregnanediol values.

2. Abnormalities of Type

Qualitative abnormalities in the amount or duration of menstrual flow are often the result of organic changes, in contrast to the abnormalities of rhythm. The most common of these disorders are hypermenorrhea, or excessive menstrual bleeding,

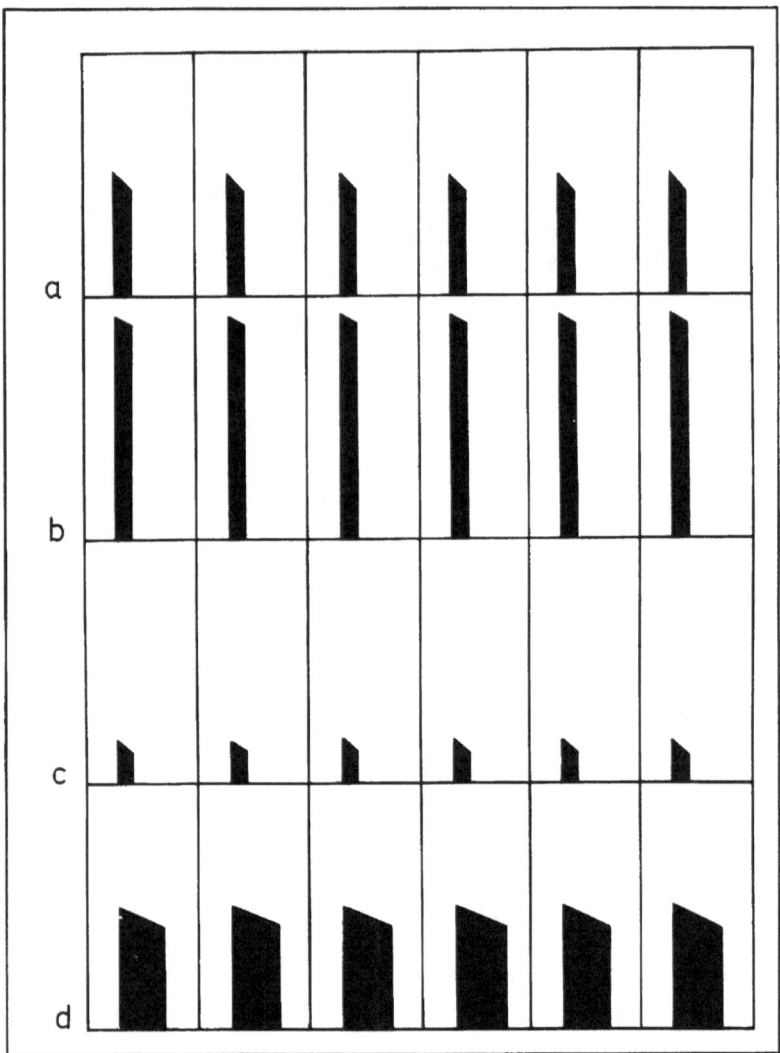

Fig. 64a–d. Abnormalities of type. **a** Eumenorrhea. **b** Hypermenorrhea. **c** Hypomenorrhea.
d Menorrhagia

and hypomenorrhea, or scanty bleeding often combined with a shortened period
of flow. These are distinguished from menorrhagia, or prolonged menstruation
(Fig. 64).

a) Hypermenorrhea

Hypermenorrhea is characterized by excessive menstrual flow with coagula,
because the fibrinolytic enzymes released from the endometrium are no longer
adequate to keep all the menstrual blood from clotting.

Pathogenesis. Hypermenorrhea is usually the result of organic changes which interfere with hemostasis, particularly a reduction of uterine contractility or, occasionally, an enlargement of the endometrial surface. Frequent causes are intramural or submucous myomas, mucosal polyps, and adenomyosis; inflammatory pelvic disease and anatomic anomalies are occasionally responsible.

Diagnosis. The diagnosis rests upon the history, a thorough clinical examination, and a hemoglobin determination to check for anemia. Fractional curettage is often useful both diagnostically and therapeutically. Other studies, particularly hormone assays, are of little value.

Treatment. Treatment must be directed mainly toward the cause. If operative measures are unnecessary, medical treatment with a gestagen-base oral contraceptive such as Stediril (Wyeth), Eugynon (Schering), or Ovulen (Searle) may be tried.

b) Hypomenorrhea

Hypomenorrhea is the term applied to scanty menstrual flow lasting only 1–2 days, and sometimes only a few hours.

Pathogenesis. In contrast to other types of abnormalities hypomenorrhea is usually caused by endocrine disturbances, particularly those which are also responsible for oligomenorrhea (which is often accompanied by hypomenorrhea) and the secondary amenorrhea that occasionally develops from it. Sometimes hypomenorrhea is observed after endometrial atrophy following the long-term use of oral contraceptives, as well as after overvigorous curettage.

Diagnosis. Special investigations are usually unnecessary in practice; hormone assays are indicated only if hypogonadism or sterility is present.

Treatment. Mild cases require no special therapy. In anovular sterility, treatment corresponds to that for amenorrhea (see p 81). If atrophy or traumatic lesions of the endometrium are present, long-term estrogen therapy may be tried; sequential estrogen-base preparations such as Cyclacur (Schering) and Trisequens (Novo) are particularly suited for this purpose.

c) Menorrhagia

Menorrhagia is the term applied to menstrual flows lasting more than 7 but less than 14 days. More prolonged flows are classified as menometrorrhagia. The quantity may be normal or increased; heavy bleeding may cause anemia.

Pathogenesis. As in hypermenorrhea, the cause is usually organic.

Diagnosis. The diagnosis is based mainly on the gynecologic examination. Hormone studies are not helpful.

Treatment. In the absence of associated conditions requiring treatment, the best approach is the use of an oral contraceptive or related preparations such as Progylut (Schering) or Sistometril (Ciba).

3. Acyclic Bleeding

Acyclic bleeding, or metrorrhagia, is an aberration of the menstrual pattern in which bleeding occurs outside the regular intervals. It may be dysfunctional or organic in origin.

Pathogenesis. Metrorrhagia in the form of irregular intermenstrual or prolonged bleeding (Fig. 65e) may be organic (e. g., endometrial carcinoma) or dysfunctional in origin. Such functional disorders are particularly common in adolescents and premenopausal women (see p 93). The cause usually lies in persistence of the unruptured follicle before the establishment of regular menstruation or after its cessation. The sustained influence of estrogen leads to overgrowth of the endometrium varying in degree from an exaggerated proliferative phase to cystic glandular hyperplasia (Fig. 66), in which case breakthrough bleeding will eventually occur.
Regular pre- and postmenstrual bleeding (Fig. 65c, d) has a dysfunctional origin in many cases. Premenstrual staining may result from an inadequate luteal phase with a premature fall of estrogen and progesterone production. On the other hand, postmenstrual staining occurs when regression of the corpus luteum is delayed. The result is prolonged progesterone secretion, often evidenced by a slight sustained elevation of basal body temperature and progesterone secretion, which leads to delayed shedding of the endometrium. By comparison, true intermenstrual bleeding (Fig. 65b), is an almost physiological event which occurs at the time of ovulation and is usually of very short duration. It is probably caused by the postovulatory fall of estrogen (see p 49) and can thus be regarded as a meager withdrawal flow.

Diagnosis. Because serious organic causes often cannot be ruled out, fractional curettage is necessary in almost every case. An exception is intermenstrual bleeding, which can be accurately correlated with ovulation based on the basal temperature curve or the presence of intermenstrual pain. Hormone assays are seldom helpful; histologic studies are considerably more informative.

Treatment. Dysfunctional bleeding is sometimes cured by routine diagnostic curettage. In instances of recurrence within 6 months and in young girls, an attempt should be made to arrest the bleeding hormonally with an estrogen-gestagen preparation, e. g., three to four tablets Primosiston (Schering) daily for 10 days. In

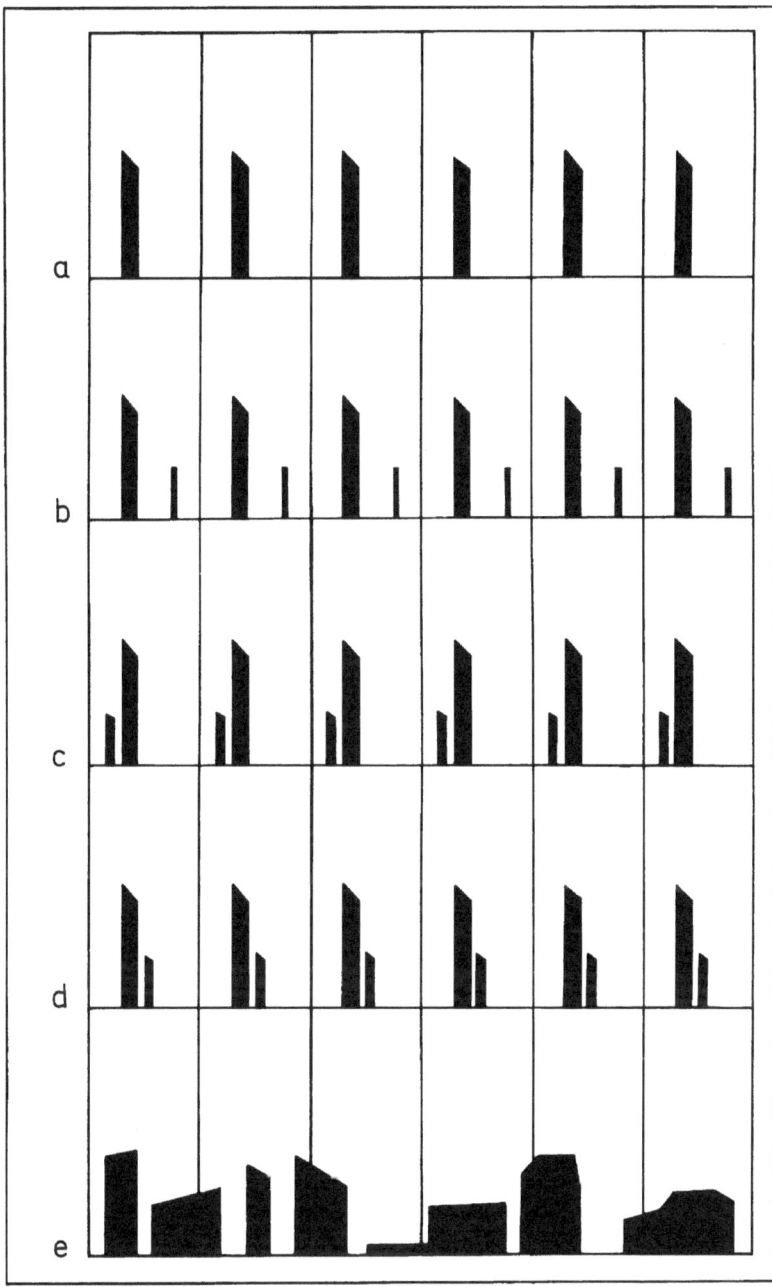

Fig. 65 a–e. Acyclic bleeding. **a** Eumenorrhea. **b** Intermenstrual bleeding. **c** Premenstrual bleeding. **d** Postmenstrual bleeding. **e** True metrorrhagia

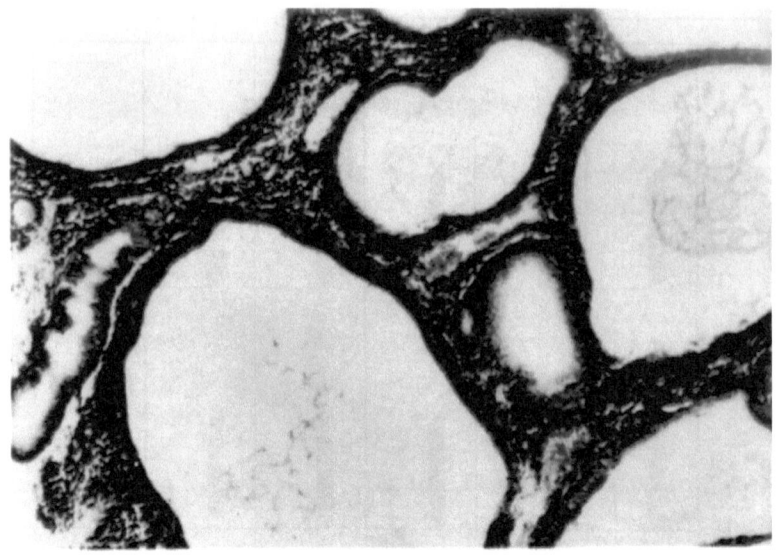

Fig. 66. Cystic glandular hyperplasia of the endometrium (x 60)

the event of further recurrences, treatment for several months with a gestagen-base oral contraceptive such as Eugynon (Schering), Stediril (Wyeth), or Ovulen (Searle) is recommended.

Premenstrual bleeding may be treated by administering gestagens, e. g., 5–10 mg Orgametril (Organon) or Primolut N (Schering), daily from cycle day 21 through 26. Postmenstrual bleeding can also be treated in this way, since withdrawal of the synthetic gestagen often leads to heavy, complete withdrawal bleeding. If the patient does not wish to conceive, good results are also achieved in both cases with oral contraceptives.

Ovulatory bleeding does not require treatment. If intermenstrual bleeding causes the patient apprehension or inconvenience, low doses of estrogen may be taken orally on cycle days 12–16, e. g., 0.02 mg Lynoral (Organon) or Progynon C (Schering) daily.

4. Dysmenorrhea and Premenstrual Tension

a) Dysmenorrhea

Dysmenorrhea is painful menstruation with cramping and sometimes persistent lower abdominal discomfort which usually accompanies the onset of bleeding, but may precede it. Nausea, vomiting, diarrhea, headaches, and irritability may also be present. The duration of these complaints may vary from a few hours to 2 days, and in some cases the pain persists throughout the menstrual period. A large percentage of women seldom suffer from painful menstruation, but in about 10% the symptoms are so severe as to be temporarily disabling.

Pathogenesis. Dysmenorrhea may be primary or secondary, depending on its time of onset. The primary form appears during or soon after the menarche and is precipitated by emotional factors in about 90% of cases. The typical patients are leptosomatic girls or socially isolated women with schizoid traits who tend to reject their own femininity. Sexual anxieties, unhappy love affairs, and loss of the security of home are frequent factors. Job disappointments may be the precipitating factor in some cases. In other cases symptoms may represent a form of aggressive protest reaction. Organic causes are decidedly less important than psychogenic ones. Uterine hypoplasia, in particular, has been overdiagnosed in painful menstruation and is, in fact, a less probable cause of dysmenorrhea than uterine malformations.

By contrast, secondary dysmenorrhea is frequently the result of organic changes. The most important is endometriosis, or the presence of ectopic endometrial implants. Characteristic complaints are associated with the intramural form, or adenomyosis, which results from simple ingrowth of the endometrium into the myometrium. Severe dysmenorrhea, often combined with dyspareunia and painful defecation, is caused by cul-de-sac and retrocervical implants. When the lesions are localized elsewhere, as in the ovary, other characteristic symptoms appear, e. g., "chocolate cysts"; tubal endometriosis is one of the most common causes of sterility in women over the age of 30 und predisposes to extrauterine pregnancy. Additional organic causes of dysmenorrhea are intramural and submucous myomas of the uterus, which can result in increased capsular tension and an increased tendency to abort. Less frequent causes are inflammatory disease, static complaints, and fixed retroflexion. Membranous dysmenorrhea, characterized by incomplete shedding of the endometrium due to an enzyme deficiency, is controversial.

Diagnosis. It is often difficult to isolate the cause of dysmenorrhea due to the presence of superimposed psychic factors. The patient's history is of prime importance; organic causes are excluded by a thorough gynecologic examination. Laparoscopy may be useful in verifying the sites of endometrial implants. Hormone assays are of no value.

Treatment. Where symptoms are mild, symptomatic treatment with analgesics and spasmolytics such as Spasmo-Cibalgin (Ciba) or Buscopan (Boehringer) may be tried. Prostaglandin synthetase inhibitors, e. g., mefenamic acid and indomethacin, are of greater benefit. Opiates are contraindicated due to rapid habituation and the risk of addiction. Psychohygienic measures, good nutrition, adequate sleep, periodic vacations, and moderate exercise are important, but true psychotherapy is indicated only in special cases. Since dysmenorrhea usually occurs in ovulatory cycles, very good results are achieved with oral contraceptives. The initial course of treatment should not exceed approximately 3 months, but longer courses must be considered if symptoms recur. Young girls generally respond well to gestagens which have a weak central action and do not inhibit ovulation, such as Duphaston

(Philips-Duphar) or Retroid (Roche), in respective doses of 10–20 and 8–12 mg per day from cycle day 5 through 25.

In endometriosis, prolonged and sometimes even permanent remission is afforded by "pseudopregnancy" hormonal therapy with increasing doses of gestagen-base ovulation inhibitors or a synthetic gestagen such as Primolut N (Schering) or Orgametril (Organon). Treatment starts several days before menstruation with a dosage of one tablet per day. The dosage is doubled after 2 weeks and tripled after another 2 weeks. After an additional 2 weeks the dosage is increased to the maintenance dose of 4–5 tablets per day. The average duration of treatment is 9 months. Excellent results are obtained with danazol (Danatrol, Winthrop), an ethisterone derivative with a strong antigonadotropic action. The dosage is 200–800 mg per day, and the rather expensive drug must be taken over a prolonged period of time. In certain cases operative treatment must be considered, as in other organic causes of dysmenorrhea.

b) Premenstrual Tension

Premenstrual tension is the term given to the physical and psychological complaints that accompany the approach of menstruation. The most prominent symptoms are painful swelling of the breasts, a sensation of fullness, pallor, edema, headaches, irritability, shifts of mood, and occasionally, genuine depression. Premenstrual water retention may be substantial. These manifestations occur as mild complaints in a great many women and may be regarded as physiologic; only about 2%–5% of cases are serious enough to warrant treatment.

Pathogenesis. Again, psychogenic factors play a significant causal role; the patients are often emotionally unstable and neurotic. Hormonal events are also a factor, since premenstrual tension is, as a rule, restricted to ovulatory cycles. However, the estrogen and progesterone levels do not differ significantly from normal values. According to one hypothesis, the substantial fluid retention is caused by increased aldosterone secretion under the influence of progesterone on the one hand, and by emotional stress on the other. An increase of vasopressin secretion has also been postulated.

Diagnosis. Special investigations are unnecessary. The diagnosis is based upon subjective complaints and clinical findings. Hormone assays are pointless.

Treatment. The principal measure is edema control through sodium restriction during the second half of the cycle, combined with a diuretic such as Lasix (Hoechst) or Hygroton (Geigy). Hormonal therapy in the form of oral contraceptives may be tried for a few months if desired; even gestagens administered during the second cycle half – e. g., 10 mg Primolut N (Schering) from cycle day 16 through 25 – are often highly effective. In severe cases, psychotherapy may be considered.

II. Amenorrhea

Amenorrhea can be classified according to a variety of criteria, as illustrated in Table 7.

Primary amenorrhea may be diagnosed if menstruation has failed to occur after the girl has passed the age of 18. This age was selected because only about 0.3% of girls experience spontaneous menarche after that time. Secondary amenorrhea is diagnosed in a patient who has menstruated but then fails to bleed for more than 3 months.

In first-degree ("generative") amenorrhea, only ovulation and luteinization are absent. Second-degree ("autonomic") amenorrhea is a much more serious disturbance in which follicular maturation, and thus estrogen production, are impaired.

Hypogonadotropic amenorrhea encompasses all serious hypothalamic-pituitary derangements. Hypergonadotropic amenorrhea is based upon an intractable failure of ovarian function, while normogonadotropic amenorrhea is due either to a uterine cause or to a mild defect of hypothalamic-pituitary regulation, such as an absence of the ovulatory LH peak.

Amenorrhea can also be classified according to local pathogenic criteria, i. e., a hypothalamic, pituitary, ovarian, uterine, or vaginal cause.

Finally, there is the physiologic form of amenorrhea normally present during childhood, pregnancy, lactation, and after menopause.

Table 7. Classification of amenorrhea

Primary amenorrhea	No spontaneous menstruation by the end of age 18
Secondary amenorrhea	Cessation of menstruation for more than 3 months
1st degree amenorrhea (generative amenorrhea)	Follicular maturation and estrogen production normal, no ovulation, no corpus luteum
2nd degree amenorrhea (autonomic amenorrhea)	Follicular maturation and estrogen production impaired, no ovulation
Hypogonadotropic amenorrhea	Hypothalamic-pituitary dysfunction, gonadotropins reduced
Normogonadotropic amenorrhea	Mild hypothalamic-pituitary or uterine dysfunction, gonadotropins within normal limits
Hypergonadotropic amenorrhea	Ovarian dysfunction, gonadotropins elevated
Physiologic amenorrhea	Childhood, prepuberty, pregnancy, lactation, postmenopausal period

1. Primary Amenorrhea

a) Hypothalamic-Pituitary Disorders

Pathogenesis. The principal feature of primary amenorrhea due to hypothalamic dysfunction is hypogonadism. Demonstrable organic changes such as aneurysms, tumors, infections, or traumata are relatively rare; the etiology is very often obscure. Lesions incurred during embryonic development have been suggested. Psychological causes are infrequent, in contrast to secondary amenorrhea (see p 79), although they are an important factor in patients with anorexia nervosa or endogenous psychoses. The picture may be further complicated by dysfunctions of other endocrine systems, such as hyper- and hypothyroidism, juvenile diabetes, or adrenogenital syndrome (see p 97).

Diagnosis. The clinical picture is that of hypogonadism, marked by underdeveloped breasts, hypoplastic genitalia, and paucity of pubic hair. Due to the lack of estrogen stimulation, there is little or no buildup of the vaginal epithelium. The gestagen test is negative, and the estrogen and gonadotropin levels are usually very low. The gonadotropin findings allow a clear differentiation from ovarian forms. In obvious cases the clomiphene test is always negative and the LH-RH test often so.

Treatment. Causal therapy is possible with human monopausal gonadotropins (see p 84), but this is a very costly and time-consuming treatment best reserved for infertile women with an urgent wish for pregnancy. Otherwise, symptomatic treatment with estrogens and gestagens, such as Cyclacur or Progylut (Schering), or a sequential oral contraceptive is recommended. It should not be started before the age of 18, because the central blocking action of these sex steroids would prevent the inception of normal pituitary-ovarian function that might still be forthcoming in cases of delayed puberty.

b) Ovarian Hypoplasia

Pathogenesis. This group is characterized chiefly by hypoplasia of the ovaries; aplasia is rare. The cause lies in developmental defects and chromosomal errors. The patients display marked hypogonadism due to estrogen deficiency.

Diagnosis. The external and internal genitalia are poorly developed, axillary and pubic hair is sparse, and the breasts are hypoplastic (Fig. 67). The basal body temperature is, of course, monophasic. The vaginal epithelium shows little or no buildup. The gestagen test is negative, estrogen levels are low, and there is a moderate to strong elevation of gonadotropins, especially FSH. The clomiphene test is negative, but the LH-RH test usually produces a further marked rise of gonadotropins. The diagnosis can be confirmed by laparoscopy and, if necessary, ovarian biopsy.

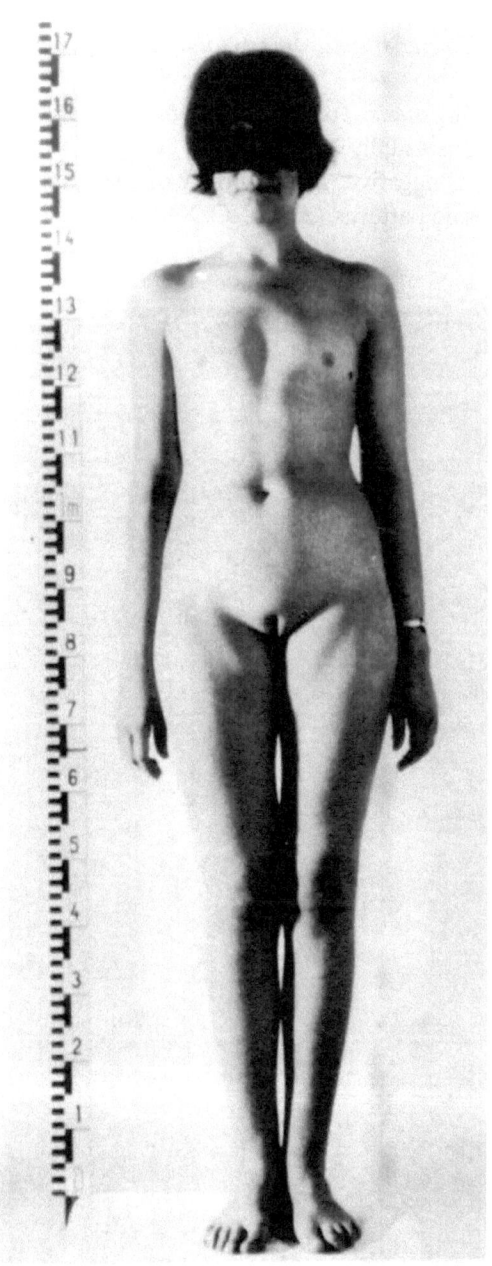

Fig. 67. Hypogonadism with primary amenorrhea in ovarian hypoplasia (22 years)

Treatment. Ovarian hypoplasia is not amenable to causal treatment, and the patient remains sterile. However, the development of secondary sex characters can be achieved by long-term estrogen replacement, e.g., 0.05–0.1 mg ethinyl estradiol per day. The concurrent or sequential administration of a gestagen, such as Sistometril (Ciba) or Progylut (Schering), is recommended. This makes it possible to evoke regular menstruation while avoiding overstimulation of the endometrium.

c) Turner's Syndrome (Gonadal Dysgenesis)

Pathogenesis. Turner's syndrome is the result of a chromosomal defect. The karyotype is usually XO, i. e., one X chromosome is absent. The sex chromatin (see p 33) is negative. In a minority of cases, structural defects of an X chromosome or mosaic patterns (e. g., XO/XX) are present, in which case the patient is chroma-

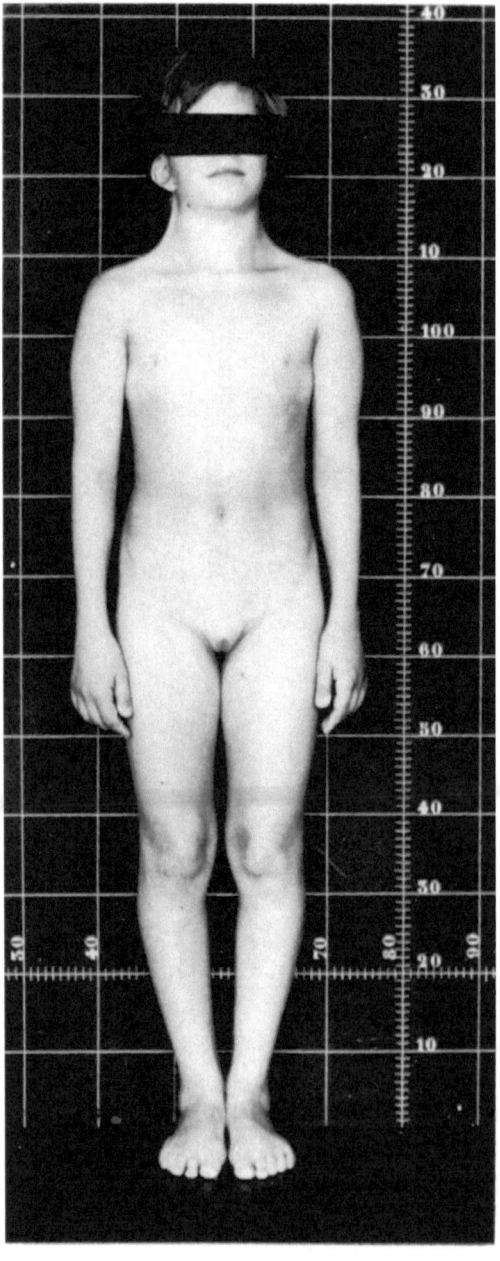

Fig. 68. Turner's syndrome (16 years)

tin-positive. The gonads are undifferentiated and of the "streak" variety, and the parenchyma is devoid of germ cells.

Diagnosis. The patients display shortness of stature and an almost complete lack of development of secondary sex characters. Webbing of the neck, cubitus valgus, and a scutiform chest with widely spaced mamillae are frequently present (Fig. 68).
As in ovarian hypoplasia, the estrogen levels are low, while the FSH values and to some extent the LH values are quite high. The gestagen and clomiphene tests are negative, but the anterior pituitary shows response to LH-RH. Laparoscopic examination reveals "streaks" in place of ovaries. The diagnosis is confirmed by chromosomal analysis, requiring special laboratory facilities.

Treatment. Treatment is at best symptomatic and is undertaken in accordance with the guidelines given above for ovarian hypoplasia.

d) Testicular Feminization

Pathogenesis. Testicular feminization is the complete form of male pseudohermaphrodism, i. e., the gonads and chromosomal sex are male. At present it is attributed to a failure of end-organ response to androgen – perhaps due to a defect in the conversion of testosterone to dihydrotestosterone – which is inherited as a sex-linked recessive trait.

Diagnosis. The patient typically appears to be a normal and well-developed female of rather tall stature. The axillary and pubic hair is scanty or absent. The external genitalia appear normal, the vagina is of varying length, ending in a blind pouch, and the uterus is absent. The gonads are always testes, which often have descended through the inguinal canal where they present as an inguinal hernia (Fig. 69). Spermiogenesis is absent, although testosterone production may equal that in a normal male. Estrogens are also formed, resulting in the marked development of female secondary sex characters. The nuclear sex is chromatin-negative, corresponding to an XY karyotype. The gonadotropins usually show a very slight increase, the estrogens are normal to slightly reduced, while the 17-ketosteroids and testosterone correspond to the normal range for males. In typical cases testicular feminization is easily diagnosed on the basis of the blind vaginal pouch and paucity of body hair with an otherwise normal female habitus. Differentiation from the more common vaginal aplasia (see p 78) is not difficult.

Treatment. If the psychosexual orientation is female, no treatment is necessary; the patient must never be informed of her "true" sex. Castration may be considered due to the risk of testicular malignancy, but this leads to deficiency symptoms which necessitate estrogen replacement. Amenorrhea and sterility cannot be cured, as the uterus is absent.

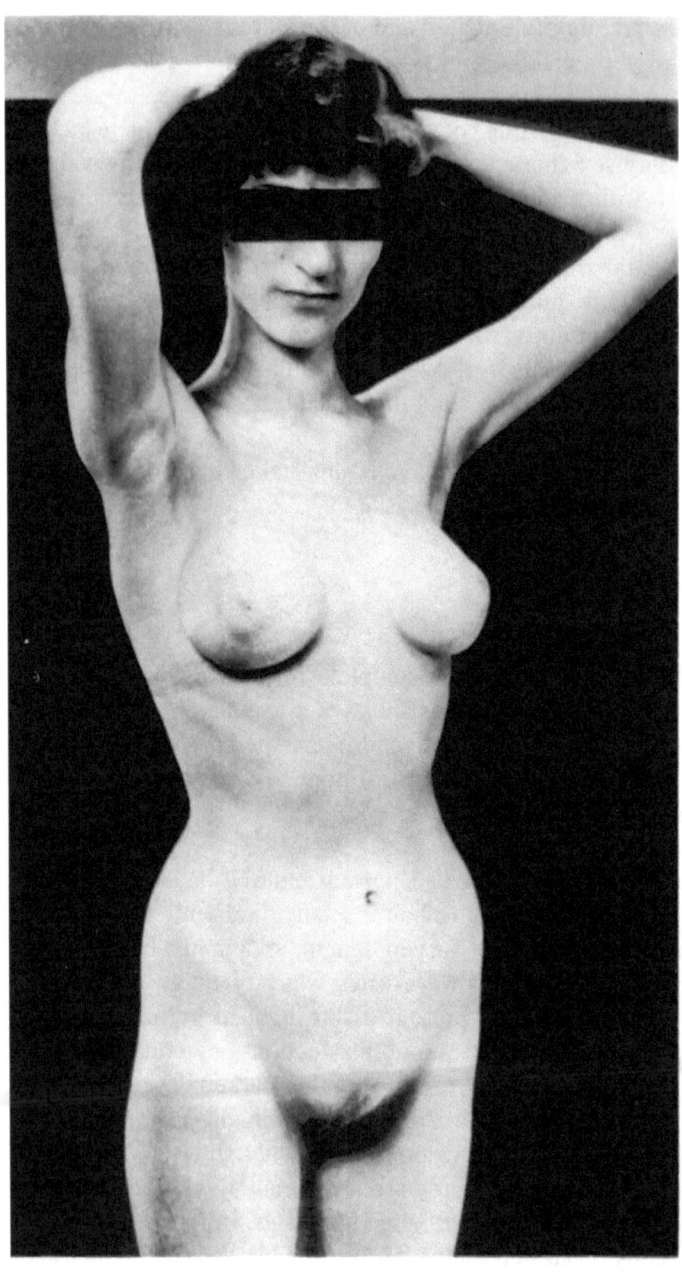

Fig. 69. Testicular feminization (20 years)

e) Mayer-Rokitansky-Kuster Syndrome

Pathogenesis. This syndrome, caused by a developmental defect of the distal Muellerian ducts, is characterized by a bipartite uterus with absence of the vagina (Fig. 70). It must be differentiated from the very rare congenital vaginal and hymenal atresias, which cause periodic, rapidly increasing pain in menstruating girls due to blockage of the menstrual flow.

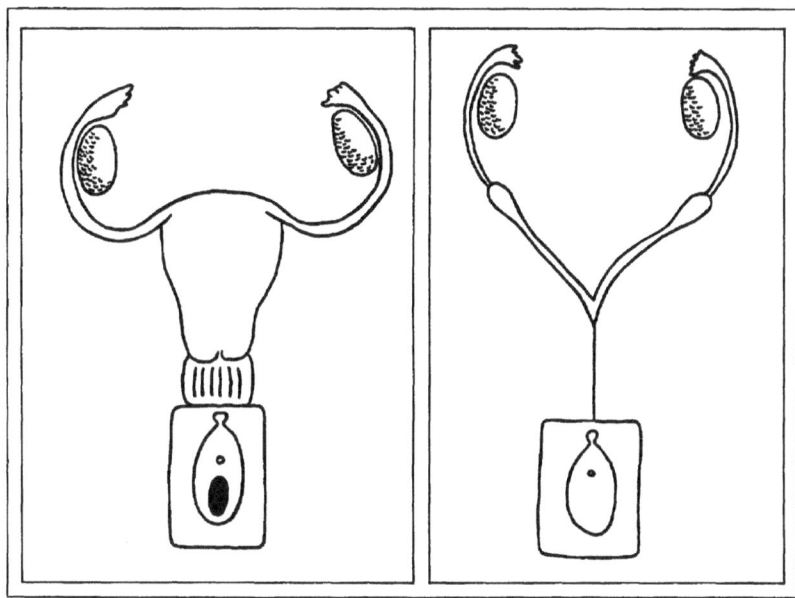

Fig. 70. Schematic drawing of the female genital tract in the normal woman (*left*) and in the Mayer-Rokitansky-Kuster syndrome (bipartite uterus with absence of vagina, *right*)

Diagnosis. The girls are quite feminine in appearance and show a completely normal external development, aside from a scantiness of body hair. The vagina is absent, while the uterus typically forms a bipartite, cordlike structure. The ovaries appear normal but are situated more superiorly than usual. Often renal anomalies are also present. The basal body temperature usually shows biphasic cycles, with normal follicular maturation, ovulation, and luteinization. The hormonal patterns correspond entirely to those in the normal woman, and the chromosomal sex is female. The diagnosis is established by careful gynecologic examination with vaginal cannulation, performed under anesthesia if necessary. Laparoscopy is indicated in doubtful cases.

Treatment. Treatment is operative, consisting of vaginal reconstruction to enable intercourse. Since the artificial vagina has a tendency to shrink, the operation should be undertaken shortly before the anticipated assumption of regular sexual activity. Of course amenorrhea and sterility cannot be corrected in these patients, due to the lack of a functional uterus.

2. Secondary Amenorrhea

a) Central Disturbances

Pathogenesis. Emotional factors play perhaps the greatest role in the origin of secondary amenorrhea. Psychogenic conflicts of all types, familial and occupational stresses, tests, marital discord, sexual problems, fear of pregnancy, and changes of environment can all produce amenorrheal symptoms. The disruption of menstruation by travel abroad or by imprisonment is particularly well known.

A special case is anorexia nervosa, a psychoneurosis characterized by aversion to eating with consequent emaciation (Fig. 71). It is usually the result of environmental problems, especially as regards the patient's relationship to her parents. An equally dramatic form of psychogenic amenorrhea is pseudocyesis, or false pregnancy. Owing to an exaggerated fear of or longing for pregnancy, the patient

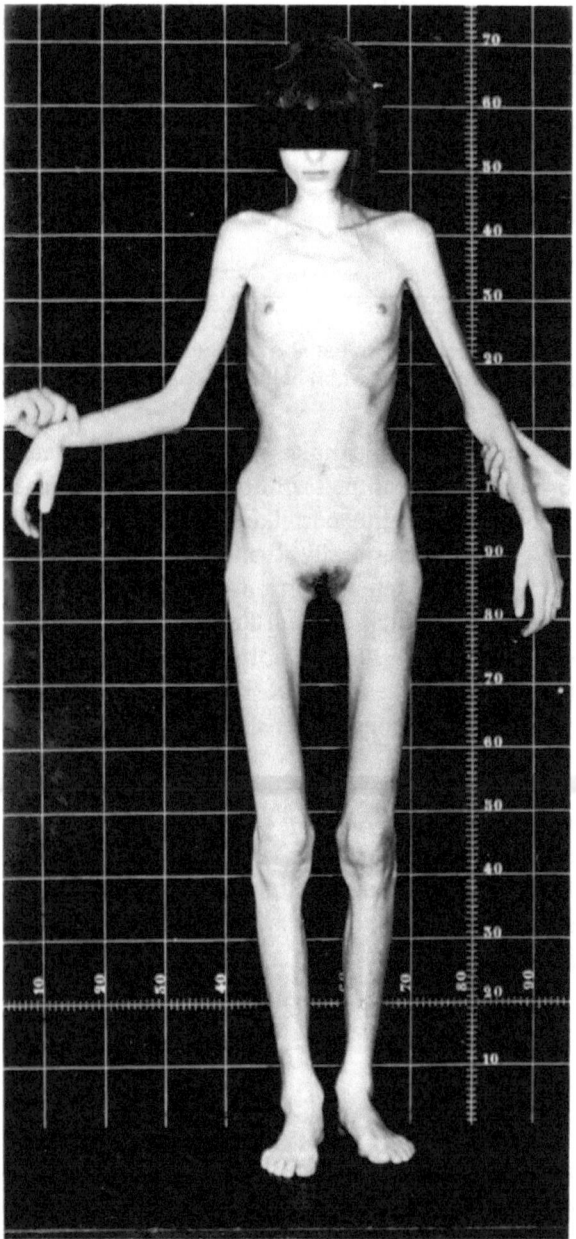

Fig. 71. Extreme emaciation in anorexia nervosa (14 years)

develops all the subjective signs including substantial weight gain, the appearance of striae, breast enlargement, and the perception of fetal movements.

Besides these psychoreactive forms, secondary amenorrhea may also occur in true psychoses and particularly in endogenous depression.

A relatively common form of secondary amenorrhea is the "oversuppression syndrome" that may follow the use of oral contraceptives. It is caused by excessive central inhibition, which tends to occur mainly after the use of gestagen-base preparations and in women with antecedent menstrual irregularity. Organic changes in the CNS, such as inflammatory processes, tumors such as craniopharyngeomas, and cranial traumata are much less common causes of amenorrhea.

Diagnosis. The patient's history and clinical examination are of greatest importance. The basal temperature curve is always monophasic due to the absence of ovulation. Estrogen and gonadotropin levels are within or slightly below normal limits; the progesterone levels are always low. The gestagen test is usually positive, as are the clomiphene and LH-RH tests. Thyroid and adrenocortical function are normal, except in anorexia nervosa and organic changes in the region of the diencephalon.

Treatment. The past 12 years have brought important breakthroughs in the treatment of these anovulatory forms of amenorrhea. Still, the medical therapy of these disorders requires considerable experience and should be left to the specialist in many cases.

The simplest measure is the cyclic administration of non-ovulation-inhibiting estrogen-gestagen combinations, such as Cyclacur (Schering). In normogonadotropic forms of secondary amenorrhea, steroids with a weak hypothalamic-stimulating action such as Retroid (Roche) (Fig. 72) have proved effective. This preparation is given in a dosage of one to three tablets of 4 mg daily for 10 days, and then from cycle day 16 through 25 once a cycle is established (Fig. 73). Ovulation occurs in only about 20% of cases, but regular menstruation is nearly always achieved. Often a normal cycle is obtained after a few months' treatment.

If the patient also wishes to conceive, more potent ovulation-inducing agents must be employed. Most suitable are the nonsteroidal cyclofenil (Fig. 74a), available commercially as Fertodur (Schering) or Sexovid (Ferrosan), and the chloro-

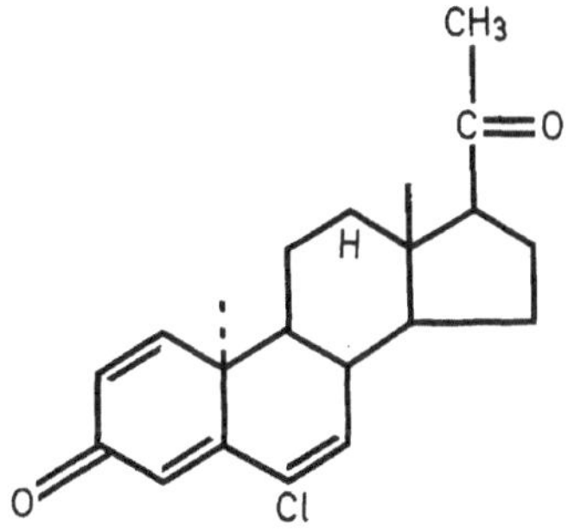

Fig. 72. Structural formula of trengestone (Retroid, Roche)

81

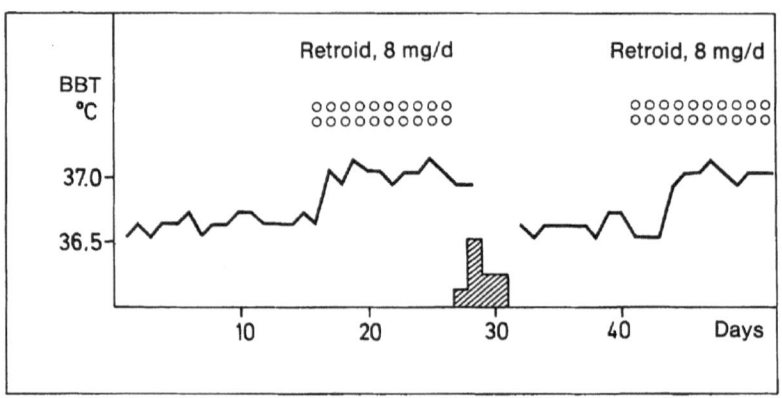

Fig. 73. Induction of ovulation with Retroid (Roche) in secondary amenorrhea

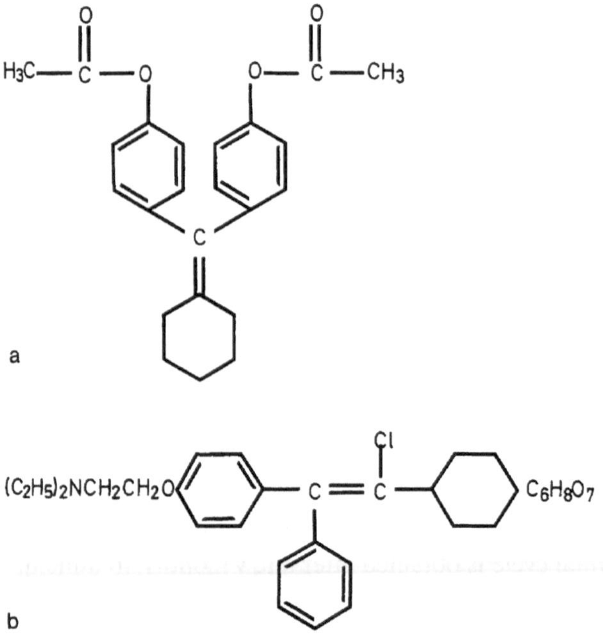

a

b

Fig. 74. a Structural formula of cyclofenil (Fertodur, Schering; Sexovid, Ferrosan). **b** Structural formula of clomiphene (Clomid, Merrell)

trianisene derivative clomiphene citrate, Clomid (Merrell) (Fig. 74b). Both agents act centrally as competetive estrogen antagonists, thereby promoting the release of pituitary gonadotropins, particularly LH. However, good results are obtained only if endogenous estrogen production is adequate, i. e., only with a positive gestagen test (see p 54). Fertodur is administered in an average dose of three tablets of 200 mg daily for 5 days, or for 10 days in resistant cases. Preferably, treatment is instituted on the 5th day of uterine bleeding evoked by 20 mg/day Primolut N

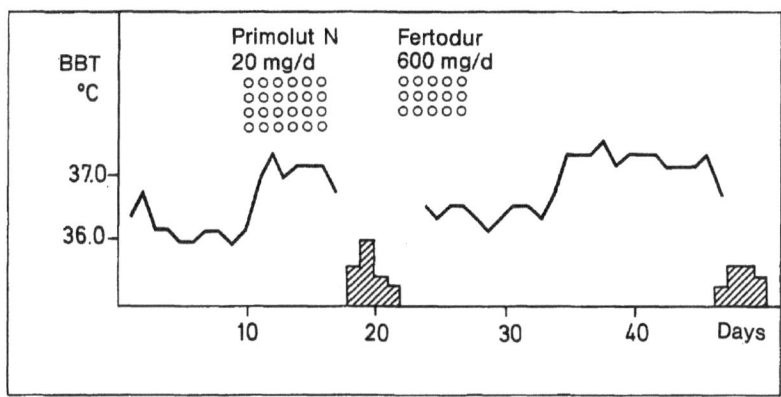

Fig. 75. Induction of ovulation with Fertodur (Schering) in secondary amenorrhea

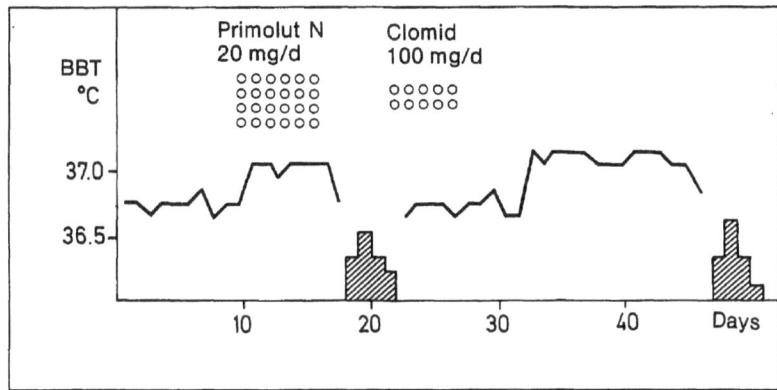

Fig. 76. Induction of ovulation with Clomid (Merrell) in secondary amenorrhea

(Schering) for 6 days, or by one ampule of Primosiston (Schering) administered intramuscularly (Fig. 75). This generally will induce ovulation between the 9th and 15th day of treatment. Unless pregnancy supervenes, menstruation will occur between about the 20th and 30th day of treatment. Fertodur is then started again on day 5.

If the cycle is anovulatory and menstruation fails to occur, gestagens are again administered to induce bleeding. Patients should be examined regularly for signs of excessive ovarian stimulation with consequent cyst formation. The ovulation rates vary from 25% to 50%, and the pregnancy rate is about 20%.

Clomid is administered in basically the same manner. The initial dosage is 50 mg daily for 5 days, which may be increased to 100–150 mg per day if results are inadequate. As with Fertodur, treatment is started on the 5th day of a spontaneous or induced menstrual flow (Fig. 76). In over 50% of cases, ovulation will occur between days 9 and 18. Again, regular examinations for signs of hyperstimulation are indicated. If ovulation is not achieved even with high doses of Clomid, then the

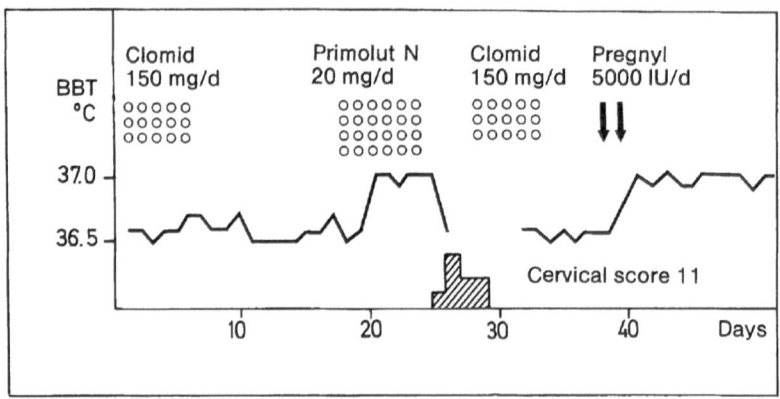

Fig. 77. Induction of ovulation with Clomid (Merrell) and HCG (Pregnyl, Organon; Primogonyl, Schering) in secondary amenorrhea

cervical mucus should be examined daily for estrogenic effect starting on about the 12th day of treatment (see p 28). When the cervical score (see p 32) reaches 10 or more, 5000–10,000 IU HCG (Pregnyl, Organon; Primogonyl, Schering) can be administered intramuscularly on 2–3 consecutive days, with close monitoring of the adnexa (Fig. 77). This will enhance the inadequate LH peak, thereby stimulating ovulation from the mature follicle. The ovulation rate then increases to 60%–70% and the pregnancy rate to 30%–40%.

If the patient still fails to ovulate, treatment with human menopausal gonadotropins (HMG) as indicated in the hypogonadotropic form of primary amenorrhea with a negative gestagen test (see p 54) must be considered. These gonadotropins are very expensive extracts of postmenopausal urine which are available commercially as Pergonal (Serono) or Humegon (Organon). Ordinarily one to four ampules, each containing 75 IU FSH and LH, are administered intramuscularly daily for about 10 days, followed by 5000–10,000 IU HCG (Pregnyl, Organon; Primogonyl, Schering; Profasi, Serono) given intramuscularly on 2–3 consecutive days (Fig. 78). During the first phase of treatment, one or more follicles are stimulated to mature; sufficient maturation can be verified by examining the cervical mucus and vaginal smear for estrogenic effect, as well as by daily estrogen assays if feasible. Monitoring of follicular growth can also be done echographically if equipment and experience permit. The actual induction of ovulation with HCG is attempted only when the cervical score (see p 32) is 10 or more; it is even better if the serum estradiol has reached 500–800 pg/ml. Patients should be closely supervised during treatment, not only because the gonadotropin dosage must be adjusted according to response, but also to avoid hyperstimulation, which is very dangerous in these patients and may lead to large cysts or multiple pregnancies with poor prognosis. Given experience and suitable patient selection, the ovulation rate is 80%–90% and the pregnancy rate 40%–50%.

Treatment with releasing hormones is still experimental (see p 2) and, for the time being, is considered only in very special cases.

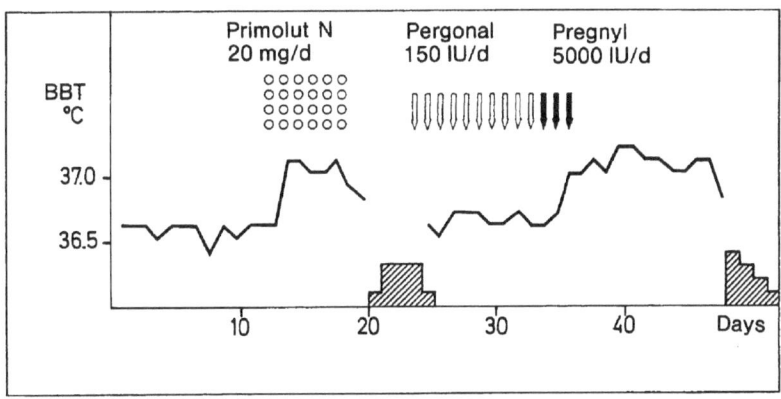

Fig. 78. Induction of ovulation with HMG (Pergonal 500, Serono; Humegon, Organon) and HCG (Pregnyl, Organon; Primogonyl, Schering; Profasi, Serono) in primary amenorrhea

b) Amenorrhea-Galactorrhea Syndrome

This includes syndromes in which the menstrual disturbance is accompanied by pathologic lactation.

Pathogenesis. The principal defect is an excessive secretion of prolactin, which probably exerts an inhibitory effect both on central control mechanisms and directly at the ovarian level. When it occurs postpartum, the phenomenon is also called the Chiari-Frommel syndrome, after its first describers; otherwise it is known as the Forbes-Albright syndrome. In most cases the common denominator is a prolactinoma of the pituitary.

Diagnosis. Following breast examination, which is always indicated, the physician looks for signs of progressive involution of the genital organs. Large pituitary tumors are excluded by the absence of associated symptoms, such as headaches, and hemianopsia; a tomographic survey of the sella turcica is also helpful.
The basal temperature curve is monophasic, the gonadotropins and estrogens are usually very low, and the gestagen test may be negative. In the absence of organic changes in the pituitary region and in cases of microadenomas, the prolactin levels show a moderate increase, while prolactinomas usually cause excessive elevation (see p 48).

Treatment. The treatment of visible pituitary adenomas is operative removal, which today is usually done transsphenoidally. If the sella is unremarkable, the condition can be effectively controlled with bromocriptin (Parlodel, Sandoz), a semisynthetic ergotamine derivative. The average dosage is three half-tablets of 2.5 mg per day, which may be doubled in resistant cases. Although ovulatory cycles usually are quickly established and galactorrhea relieved, the regimen should be maintained for several cycles. In many cases conception will occur, at which time the medication is discontinued.

c) Sheehan's Syndrome

Pathogenesis. This rare form of postpartum pituitary necrosis is a sequela of complicated deliveries with excessive uterine bleeding and shock; it is the result of spasms, microthrombosis, and ischemia of the anterior lobe.

Diagnosis. Usually the initial symptom is an inability to lactate, later followed by amenorrhea and the loss of pubic and axillary hair and lateral portions of the eyebrows (Fig. 79). The skin loses its pigment and acquires an alabasterlike color and texture. The patient becomes lethargic and prone to hypoglycemia, dizziness, and chills. Some cases progress to full panhypopituitarism with a complete loss of anterior pituitary hormones and marked psychological changes.
The gonadotropin levels are low and there is a marked estrogen deficiency, resulting in a negative gestagen and clomiphene test. The pituitary response to LH-RH is poor. Adrenocortical and thyroid function may also be affected to varying degrees.

Treatment. The hormonal adjustments are complicated and should be undertaken with the advice of an experienced endocrinologist, at least when evidence of panhypopituitarism is present. From a gynecologic standpoint, the primary therapy is estrogen replacement; if a regular cycle is desired, an estrogen-gestagen preparation such as Progylut (Schering) or a sequential oral contraceptive (Ovanon, Ercopharm) is prescribed. In patients desiring pregnancy, the only recourse is the use of costly human menopausal gonadotropins (see p 84); however, this can succeed only after adequate stimulative therapy of other pituitary target glands and the long-term treatment of uterine hypoplasia with estrogens.

d) Premature Menopause

Pathogenesis. The premature failure of ovulation before the age of 40 is not entirely uncommon. The etiology is unclear but may involve vascular processes linked to the genetic makeup. The course is essentially that of the normal climacteric, except that it occurs years prematurely: The periods first become irregular and then cease altogether, accompanied by hot flushes and other deficiency symptoms.

Diagnosis. The early clinical findings are somewhat uncharacteristic, but the high level of gonadotropins and low estrogen values help to establish the diagnosis.

Treatment. Causal therapy is not possible due to the failure of follicular maturation and thus of autonomic ovarian function. Replacement therapy with estrogens is useful for symptomatic relief (see p 93). Young patients who for psychological reasons wish to continue menstruating regularly can be treated with a sequential preparation such as Progylut (Schering), Ovanon (Ercopharm), or Trisequens (Novo).

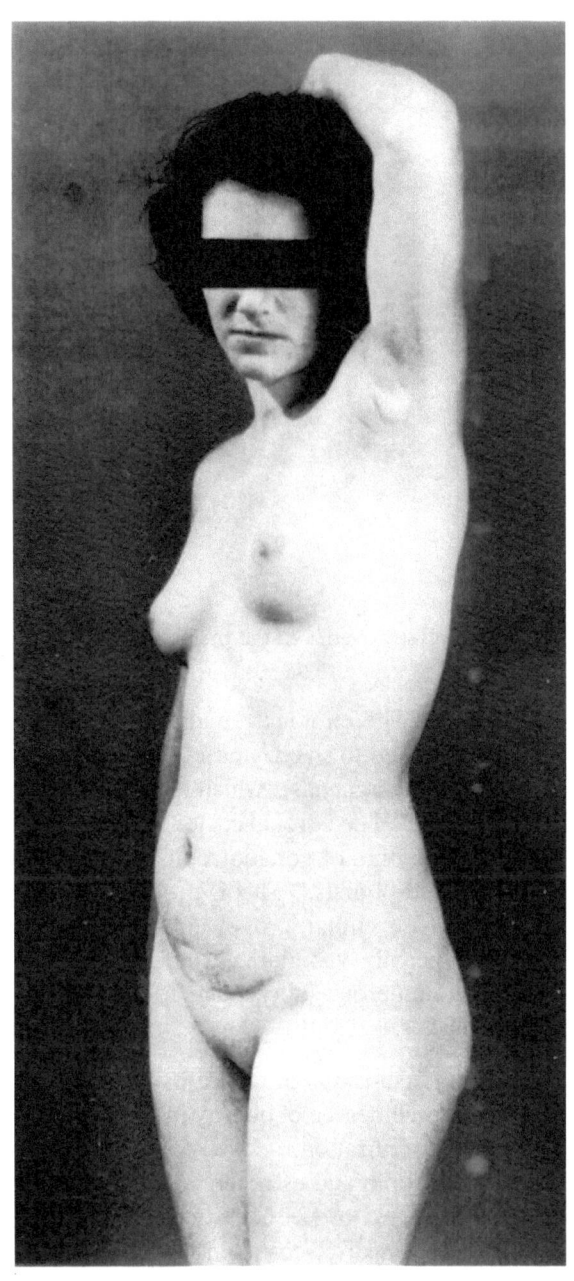

Fig. 79. Sheehan's syndrome (29 years)

e) Stein-Leventhal Syndrome

The Stein-Leventhal syndrome, or bilateral polycystic ovaries, is a special, somewhat vaguely circumscribed clinical entity which can lead to secondary amenorrhea or oligomenorrhea. Statistically, it occurs in 1%–4% of all women, though this incidence is naturally much higher among sterile patients. Only about one-fourth of patients remain fertile without treatment.

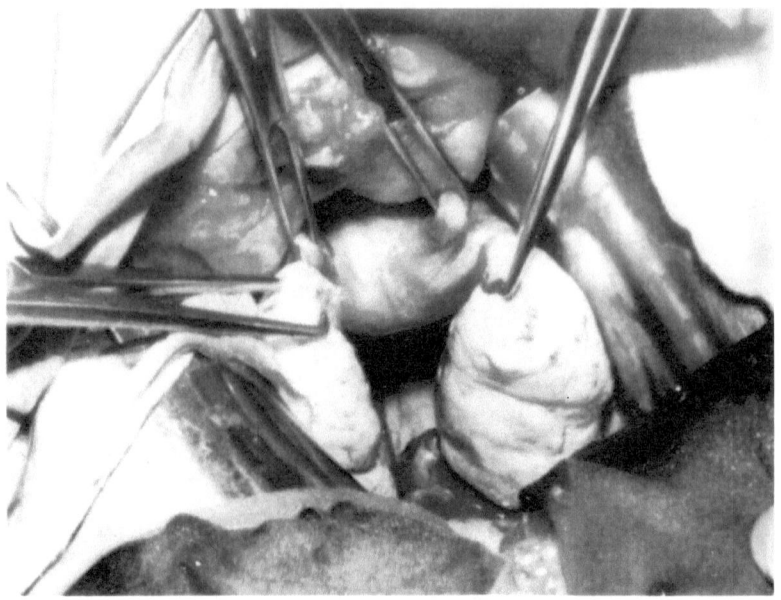

Fig. 80. Polycystic ovaries in the Stein-Leventhal syndrome

Pathogenesis. The etiology remains disputed. Based on all available results, it is apparently linked to an enzymatic defect of ovarian steroid biosynthesis, especially of 3β-OH-dehydrogenase, which leads to an increased production of androgens in the ovary itself. The adrenal cortex may also be involved. There is often a disturbance in the rhythm of gonadotropin secretion, with an excessive release of LH in closely spaced "bursts." This is probably responsible for the true cardinal symptom of Stein-Leventhal: grossly enlarged, polycystic ovaries, typically with a grayish-white, heavily vascularized capsule (Fig. 80). The histologic picture shows sometimes numerous subcapsular follicular cysts and an abnormal abundance of atretic follicles.

Diagnosis. Hirsutism is observed in about 70% of patients, amenorrhea in about 50%, and some degree of obesity in 40% (Fig. 81). About 20% of patients display true signs of virilization.
The gonadotropin and estrogen values are variable and not characteristic. Sometimes an elevation of LH activity can be found. An increase of urinary 17-ketosteroids and 17-hydroxycorticoids is observed in about a third of cases; the androsterone and etiocholanolone fractions, in particular, show an increase. The plasma testosterone levels generally are above 1 ng/ml (see p 53); the serum androstenedione is also elevated.
The diagnosis and differentiation from hyperfunction of the adrenal cortex, as in acquired adrenogenital syndrome (see p 87), rest mainly upon the demonstration of polycystic ovaries. They may be palpable, but their presence can be verified only by laparoscopy and biopsy. In special cases the combined dexamethasone-HCG test (see p 61) may be helpful.

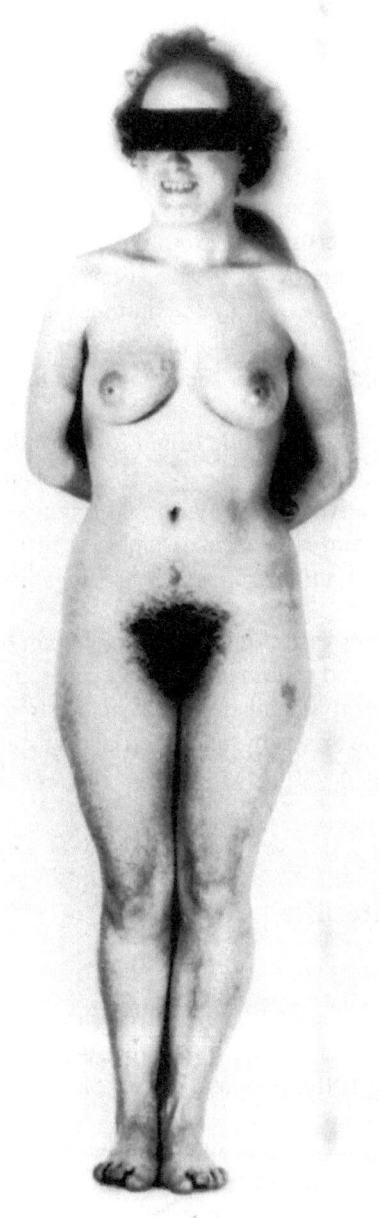

Fig. 81. Virilization in the Stein-Leventhal syndrome (31 years)

Treatment. In pronounced cases the treatment of choice is bilateral wedge resection of the ovaries. This qualitatively alters the impaired ovarian steroid biosynthesis to the extent that normal hypothalamic-gonadal interaction can be achieved. Menstrual rhythm is restored in about 80% of patients, and about 60% become pregnant; hirsutism is improved only sporadically. Unfortunately, the recurrence rate is rather high. The syndrome may also be treated medically with antiandrogens (see p 96). In patients wishing to conceive, ovulation should be induced with Fertodur (Schering), Clomid (Merrell) or HMG (see p 81), though caution is advised due to the high risk of cyst formation in these patients.

f) Intrauterine Changes

The most common form of intrauterine damage is Asherman's syndrome, which usually occurs as a result of overvigorous postpartum or postabortal curettage. Due to the loss of the basal layer, there is a failure of endometrial regeneration, while the ovarian cycle continues unchanged. Damage may also result from manual separation of the placenta and other intrauterine manipulations, as well as from inflammation such as tubercular endometritis.

Diagnosis. A uterine origin for secondary amenorrhea is usually suggested by the patients' history. The gynecologic examination and hormone workup are seldom informative. Despite a biphasic temperature curve, good buildup of the vaginal epithelium, and normal values for serum gonadotropins and sex steroids, both the gestagen and estrogen test are negative, and this establishes the diagnosis.

Treatment. Intrauterine adhesions can be separated by curette, sound, or hysteroscope, and mucosal remnants can sometimes be stimulated to proliferate by the long-term administration of high estrogen doses. Satisfactory results are achieved in some cases by endometrial transplantation, but in general the prognosis is uncertain.

III. Sterility

Infertility is not necessarily the result of endocrinopathy, yet both physician and patient very often make this presumption. We shall therefore present a brief survey of the principal causes of sterility, their recognition, and treatment.

Causes. Of all marriages, 10%–15% are childless. Thus, the problem of sterility is common and, for many women, very painful. Approximately 30%–40% of barren marriages result from sterility of the male, 35%–45% from sterility of the female, while 10–20% have no demonstrable cause. Some 40% of female sterility cases are due to hormonal disorders, 30% to tubal abnormalities, and 10%–20% to cervical factors. The remaining cases have rarer causes or remain unexplained. Psychogenic factors can also play a role, particularly in disturbances of tubal motility which interfere with ovum transport.

Diagnosis. The figures cited above suggest the most effective program of investigation (Table 8). It is instituted only if pregnancy has failed to occur within one year

Table 8. Evaluation of infertility

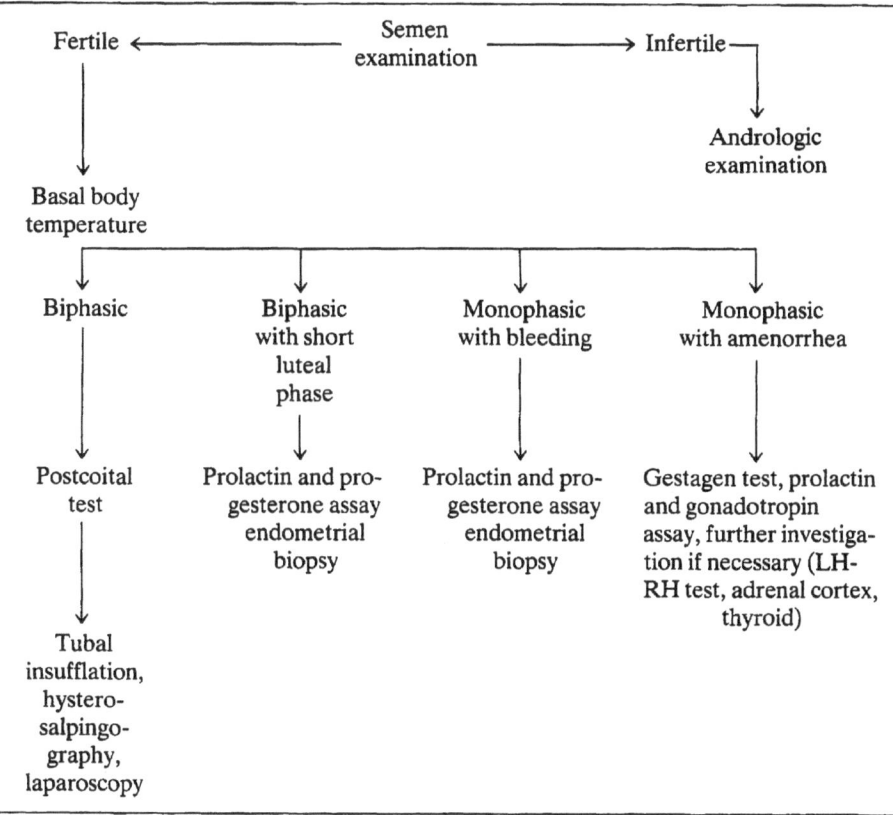

after the assumption of regular sexual intercourse without the use of contraceptives. First the male factor must be excluded by a semen analysis (see p 37). If poor results are obtained on repeated analysis, the patient is referred to an experienced andrologist for further consultation. In the case of the woman, a thorough history is taken, followed by a general and gynecologic examination (see p 20). Even with apparently regular cycles, a basal temperature record should be kept for at least 1 month (see p 20) as a means of recognizing failure of ovulation or luteal deficiency (see p 21), which is quite common. In the event of anovulation, further menstrual studies are done, including prolactin assays; a short luteal phase, on the other hand, necessitates endometrial biopsy (see p 32) and progesterone determination. In every case tubal patency must be tested by insufflation, hysterosalpingraphy, or laparoscopy (see p 40). Finally, the postcoital test (see p 37) is necessary to evaluate compatibility conditions, even if the semen analysis is normal.

Treatment. Once the diagnosis is established, treatment can begin. The infertile male may be treated operatively or with androgens, clomiphene, or human gonadotropins, depending on the findings. However, the prognosis is not very favorable. In the female, ovulatory disturbances are often amenable to medical treatment (see p 83). Tubal impatency is correctable by microsurgery, but these operations are only promising in the hands of an experienced specialist. The situation is most difficult in cases of immunologically determined incompatibility. Occasionally, the use of a condom is prescribed for several months to effect desensitization, but results are not often favorable. Homologous artificial insemination may be successful in selected patients.

All treatments mentioned are time consuming and thus require patience and diligence on the part of all concerned. Despite this, some 25%–50% of infertile marriages can be rendered fertile with treatment.

IV. The Peri- and Postmenopausal Period

1. Deficiency Symptoms

Pathogenesis. The progressive decline of ovarian estrogen production during the climacteric and especially after menopause creates a "menopausal syndrome" in many women. It is also brought on by castration. The syndrome not only affects the hypothalamic-pituitary-ovarian axis, but also leads to functional derangements of other autonomic centers in the diencephalon. Symptoms include irritability, headaches, forgetfulness, insomnia, and depression; but the most characteristic complaint is the hot flush, which occurs in over 80% of women. It takes the form of disturbing paroxysmal hyperemia of the face, neck, chest, and hands, accompanied by a sensation of heat and sweating. The pathogenic details are unclear but may involve regulation disturbances in the region of the cervical sympathicus. Circulatory symptoms include palpitation of the heart, vertigo, and tinnitus aurium (Table 9).

Besides disturbances of endocrine origin, menopausal women often experience psychological difficulties relating mainly to changes in living habits and to aging in general. Loss of the figure, children moving away or occupational problems may be precipitating factors.

One result of the estrogen deficiency, of course, is the occurrence of organic changes such as involution of the genital organs. Dyspareunia, senile vaginitis, and urethrocystitis are expressions of these changes. After menopause, senile osteoporosis develops much more frequently than in men. There also appears to be a link between estrogen deprivation and the obesity common in this age group, although lack of exercise and increased caloric intake are primarily responsible.

In some circumstances the menopausal syndrome may considerably precede the menopausal event. The symptoms usually regress within a few years but occasionally persist to an advanced age. Both the duration and intensity of the syndrome depend strongly on the psychological makeup of the woman involved. Her education, environment, and degree of adjustment play a decisive role. Hormone assays are of little value, since subjective complaints generally are sufficient to establish the diagnosis, except in premature menopause, q. v. The gonadotropin levels are elevated and the estrogen levels reduced, but these bear no direct relation to the severity of symptoms.

Table 9. Menopausal syndrome

	Symptoms
Psychic	Shifts in mood
	Irritability
	Nervousness
	Depression
	Insomnia
	Forgetfulness
	Headaches
Vascular	Hot flushes
	Sweating
	Heart palpitation
	BP variability
	Dizziness
	Tinnitus aurium
General	Reduced ability to perform tasks
	Weight gain
	Constipation
	Osteoporosis
	Atrophy of genitalia

Treatment. In many cases treatment is essential, and estrogen is the agent of choice. Most suitable are the conjugated steroids, which have little endometrial activity and so are unlikely to cause bleeding. An example is Premarin (Ayerst), taken in a dosage of 0.625–1.25 mg cyclically for 3 weeks, followed by 1 week without its use. Patients with psychological problems may respond to Menrium (Roche), a product which combines conjugated estrogens with Librium. Furthermore, the continuous or intermittent administration of estriol (Ovestin, Organon) or estriol succinate (Synapause, Nourypharma) in an average daily dosage of 1–2 and 2–4 mg, respectively, has proved to be of great value; these preparations also cause little endometrial stimulation. In resistant cases, the combination of androgen and estrogen in the form of a depot preparation, such as Femandren (Ciba), may be considered. The intramuscular injection of a crystalline suspension has a duration of action of 3–5 weeks. In certain cases the salutary effects of the testosterone component may be accompanied by an increased libido and mild virilization.

2. Bleeding

a) Pre- and Perimenopausal Bleeding

Pathogenesis. As in juveniles (see p 68), dysfunctional bleeding in climacteric women is usually the result of a persistent unruptured follicle. In such cases the follicle develops to the tertiary or vesicular stage (see p 7), but ovulation does not occur due to the inadequacy of hypothalamic regulation. The increasing estrogenic effect causes excessive endometrial proliferation, leading after several weeks to cystic glandular hyperplasia (see p 68) (Fig. 66). In very rare cases, a granulosa cell tumor may create the same situation (see p 94). When the estrogen level falls below that required to sustain the hyperplastic endometrium, varying degrees of bleeding occur, ranging from slight staining to severe hemorrhage that may persist for weeks.

Diagnosis. Hormone assays yield little information, though estrogen levels may be somewhat elevated. Since organic changes are present in over 20% of climacteric menometrorrhagia, fractional curettage should be performed in every case. In cystic glandular hyperplasia, curettage has both a diagnostic and therapeutic role. Abnormal bleeding tends to recur in approximately two-thirds of cases, which may then be treated hormonally after malignancy is excluded. Bleeding can be effectively controlled with orally active estrogen-gestagen preparations, e. g., three to five tablets Primosiston (Schering) daily for 10 days. This regimen provokes heavy withdrawal bleeding and thus serves as a "hormonal curettage." For long-term therapy, oral contraceptives with a high gestagen content are suitable, such as Eugynon (Schering) or Ovulen (Searle). Parenteral depot preparations are less suitable, because their prolonged hormonal activity may lead to sustained, heavy withdrawal bleeding.

b) Postmenopausal Bleeding

Pathogenesis. In most cases postmenopausal bleeding is the result of organic changes. It may also be caused by cystic glandular hyperplasia due to the long-term administration of estrogen-containing preparations with considerable endometrial activity. In rare cases the estrogen source is a follicle which matures postmenopausally or an ovarian neoplasm, notably a granulosa cell tumor or a theca cell tumor. These are estrogen-producing, usually unilateral, semimalignant tumors whose volume is highly variable; they may reach an enormous size, or may be only a few millimeters in diameter and thus difficult to locate.

Diagnosis. Curettage is always indicated in postmenopausal bleeding. Further investigations depend upon histologic findings. If cystic glandular hyperplasia is discovered, all estrogen-containing ointments and tablets must be withdrawn. Moderately elevated estrogen levels in the serum or urine accompanied by an abnormally low postmenopausal level of pituitary gonadotropins are indicative of a hormone-producing ovarian tumor. In doubtful cases the diagnosis is verified by laparoscopy.

Treatment. When bleeding is from hormonal causes, uterine curettage is of therapeutic value. Exogenous estrogens must be discontinued and replaced when necessary with estriol preparations having less endometrial activity, such as Ovestin (Organon). If the diagnosis of granulosa cell tumor is established, hysterectomy and bilateral adnexectomy is indicated; postoperative irradiation may be advised in certain cases.

V. Hirsutism and Virilism

1. Hirsutism

Hirsutism is the term applied to a masculine pattern of hair growth. It may be due to constitutional factors and is particularly common in women of Mediterranean origin. It is manifested by increased hairiness of the chin, cheeks, and upper lip. The pubic hair appears masculine and may extend to the navel. There is usually a thick periareolar hair growth on the breasts, sometimes reaching beyond the sternum (Fig. 82). Excessive hair is also noted on the lower leg and forearm and occasionally on the thigh. Other signs of masculinization are absent; in particular, the voice and body contours remain feminine and there is no clitoral hypertrophy. True hirsutism is distinct from hypertrichosis, which is simply an excessive feminine hair growth.

Pathogenesis. Most cases of hirsutism are of constitutional origin and are unaccompanied by any demonstrable endocrine disturbance. This "idiopathic" form probably involves a heightened responsiveness of the receptors to the androgens

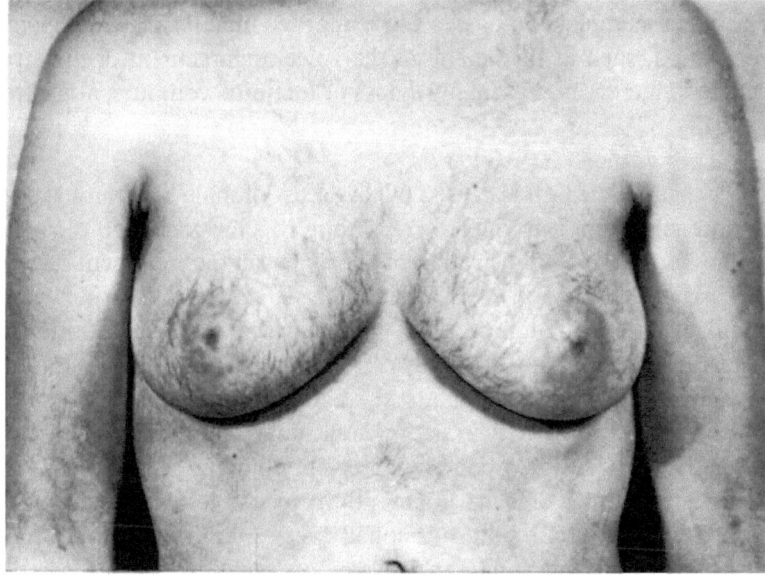

Fig. 82. Hirsutism

normally present in women. It is distinguished from ovarian hirsutism, as in the Stein-Leventhal syndrome (see p 87), and adrenal hirsutism, as encountered in latent forms of adrenocortical hyperplasia.

Diagnosis. Diagnosis begins with the patient's history and clinical examination. Determinations are then made of the urinary 17-ketosteroids or, preferably, the plasma testosterone; the serum androstenedione and dehydroepiandrosterone are also determined when necessary (see p 53). If these findings are normal and no ovarian changes are found, the hirsutism may be classified as idiopathic. However, follow-up examination after several months is mandatory. If elevated values are found, an accurate test of ovarian and adrenocortical function is indicated, as in virilization. The results may warrant further investigations, such as laparoscopy, tomography, retropneumoperitoneum, or angiography.

Treatment. It is possible today to treat hirsutism hormonally by means of antiandrogens. Cyproterone acetate (Androcur, Schering) combined with estrogens has proved to be particularly effective. The dosage is 50–100 mg daily from cycle day 5–14, combined with 0.05 mg ethinyl estradiol daily (Lynoral, Organon; Progynon C, Schering) from cycle day 5–25. A corresponding preparation has been in the trial stage for several years (SH 8.1041). The duration of treatment is at least 6–9 months, and recurrences are frequent, even with initially good results. In hirsutism from adrenal hyperplasia, prednisone or dexamethasone may be tried (see p 99). In any case, depilation with cosmetic agents should be considered.

2. Virilism

This term is employed in cases where marked hirsutism is accompanied by signs of virilization, such as deepening of the voice, enlargement of the larynx, temporal baldness, increased musculature, loss of feminine contours, and clitoral hypertrophy (Fig. 83).

Pathogenesis. Virilism is caused by an excess of male sex steroids of either ovarian or adrenal origin. Infrequently, it is an iatrogenic condition caused, for example, by the long-term administration of androgens in the treatment of cystic diseases of the breast. Virilization of ovarian origin is rare and is usually the result of an androgen-producing tumor, though it may also be associated with Stein-Leventhal syndrome in a few cases (see p 87). The principal tumor type is the androblastoma, a semimalignant, usually unilateral, solid, and occasionally cystic ovarian tumor which varies considerably in size and may not be palpable. The histologic picture is marked by large, lipoid-containing, eosinophilic interstitial cells which resemble those of the testes and are apparently responsible for the androgen production. Not all androblastomas are hormonally active, but on the other hand, other rare types of ovarian tumor can be virilizing on occasion, such as gynandroblastomas, hilus cell tumors, lipoid cell tumors, and gonadoblastomas. More common than

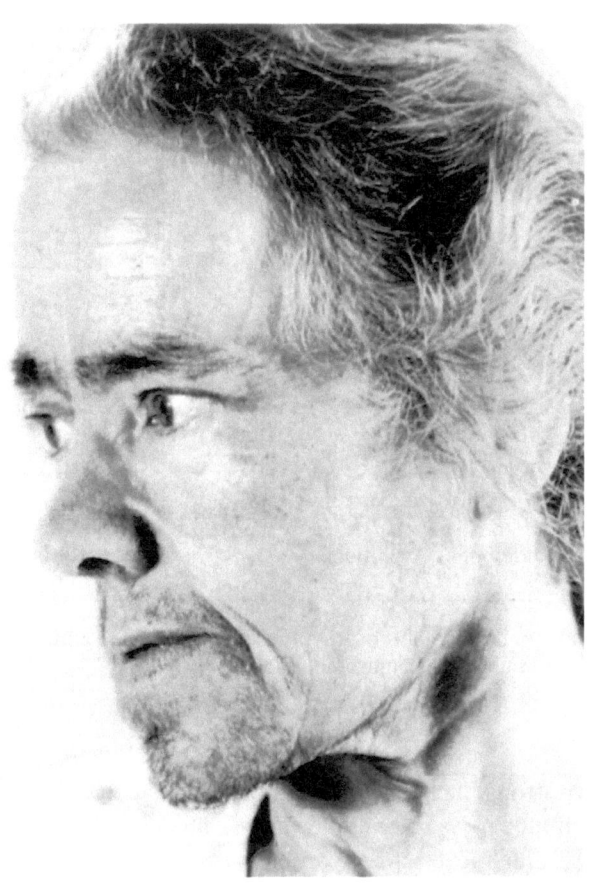

Fig. 83. Virilization in adrenal cortical adenoma (55 years)

ovarian virilization is that of adrenal origin, as seen in the acquired adrenogenital syndrome. The cause lies in hyperplasia, adenoma, or carcinoma of the adrenal cortex. The acquired adrenogenital syndrome is distinguished from the congenital adrenogenital syndrome, in which adrenal cortical hyperplasia with excessive androgen production has its onset during fetal development. It is transmitted as a recessive trait and results from a congenital defect of 21-hydroxylation or, less frequently, of 11-β-hydroxylation in the adrenal cortex. This interferes with the biosynthesis of cortisol (see Fig. 84), which leads to a compensatory increase in ACTH secretion and thus to an excessive formation of male sex steroids.

Diagnosis. The most salient clinical features are defeminization and virilization. The breasts, uterus, and vagina become atrophic, and there is oligo- or amenorrhea with marked hirsutism; the voice deepens, often temporal baldness appears, and finally the clitoris becomes hypertrophic. The basal body temperature is monophasic, the vaginal smear shows an atrophic picture, and the gonadotropins and estrogens are usually low. The 17-ketosteroids show a slight increase in Stein-Leventhal syndrome, a moderate increase in androblastoma, a moderate

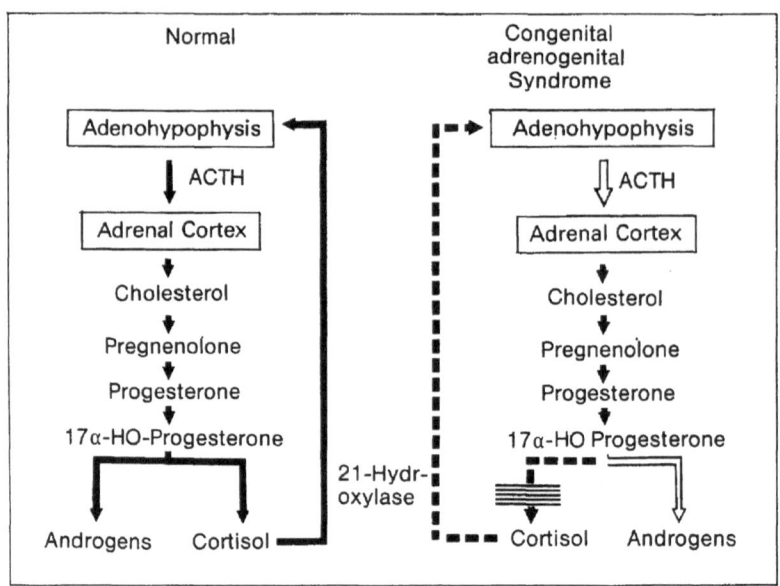

Fig. 84. Schema of the biosynthesis of cortisol and androgens in normal cases and in congenital adrenogenital syndrome

to strong increase in adrenocortical adenoma, and a very strong increase in adrenocortical carcinoma (up to 100 mg/24 h). Specific assays, moreover, reveal a very high level of dehydroepiandrosterone when the process is of adrenal origin. The plasma testosterone levels may also rise substantially, particularly in androgen-secreting ovarian tumors, when values typically occupy the range normal for males, i. e., in excess of 5 ng/ml.

Differential diagnosis is possible only with the aid of further studies. A positive dexamethasone suppression test (see p 59), a marked rise of 17-ketosteroids in response to ACTH (see p 58), and elevated pregnanetriol levels in the urine are indicative of hyperplasia or adenoma of the adrenal cortex. Further information including localization of the lesion is afforded by radiologic methods such as tomography, retropneumoperitoneum, and angiography. If suppression of high 17-ketosteroids is poor, an adrenocortical carcinoma must be suspected.

The diagnosis of congenital adrenogenital syndrome is usually made solely from the patient's history and clinical examination. In the male the virilism produces only false precocious puberty, whereas in females it causes pseudohermaphrodism with intersexual external genitalia and marked clitoral hypertrophy (Fig. 85). Untreated cases also display an acceleration of bone growth. The secondary sex characters appear between the age of 2 and 10 and, like the overall physique, become increasingly masculine. As a rule the patient does not menstruate, and the adult is entirely virile in appearance. Hormone assays again show low gonadotropin values, while the urinary 17-ketosteroids and plasma testosterone are greatly increased. The urinary estrogens may be normal or even elevated due to metabo-

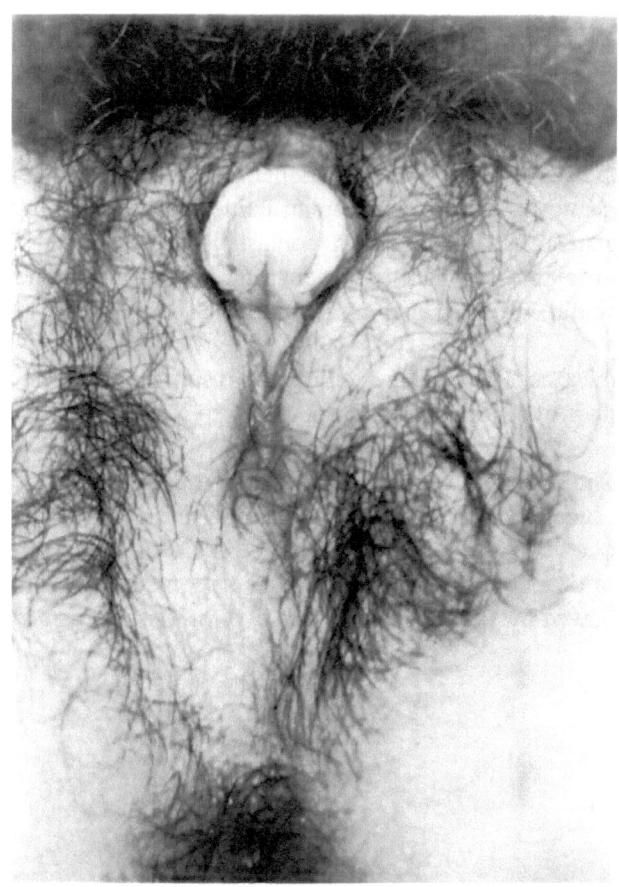

Fig. 85. Clitoral hypertrophy in congenital adrenogenital syndrome

lism of the androgens, while the plasma cortisol is reduced. The urinary 17-hydroxycorticosteroids often show a reduction as well, but this is not very specific.

Treatment. The treatment for tumors is operative removal. Androblastomas require hysterectomy with bilateral adnexectomy.

In adrenal hyperplasia, the long-term administration of prednisone is indicated to suppress excessive androgen production. Generally the dosage is 2.5–10 mg per day, adjusted according to the excretory values of 17-ketosteroids, which should remain below 10 mg/24 h. Overdosage can lead to iatrogenic Cushing syndrome.

In congenital adrenogenital syndrome, long-term treatment with glucocorticoids such as prednisone must be instituted. This will inhibit excessive ACTH secretion on the one hand, while affording cortisone replacement on the other. The dosage is critical and should be set by a specialist; for prednisone it is approximately 6 mg/m^2 body surface per day. If treatment is started very early, a completely normal development can be achieved. In many cases the patients menstruate regularly after puberty and possess normal reproductive function.

VI. Diseases of the Mammary Glands

1. Mammary Hypoplasia

Pathogenesis. Underdevelopment of the breasts (Fig. 86) is usually a constitutional variant, probably caused by an inadequate response of the parenchyma to hormonal stimuli. Mammary hypoplasia is also observed in hypogonadism from ovarian failure, in which case menstrual abnormalities and poor development of the external and internal genitalia are also seen.

Diagnosis. The clinical examination is sufficient, and hormone assays are indicated only if hypogonadism is suspected (see p 73).

Treatment. In the constitutional form, pharmacologic measures offer little prospect of success, while estrogen-containing ointments afford, at best, only transitory improvement. Better results can be achieved by the long-term cyclic administration of an estrogen-gestagen combination such as Sistometril (Ciba) for 3 weeks followed by 1 week with no usage, or of Trisequens forte (Novo). Such treatment

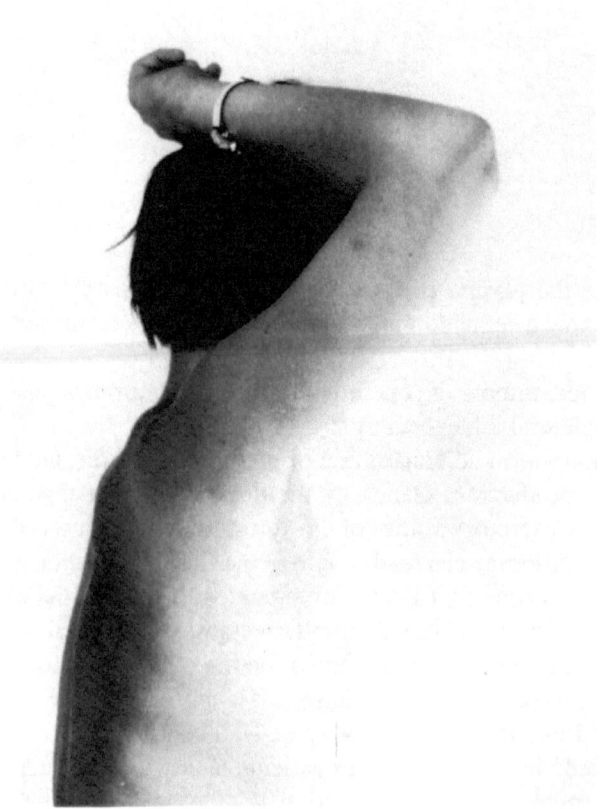

Fig. 86. Hypoplasia of the breasts (21 years)

is particularly suitable for those forms of hypogonadism in which spontaneous development can no longer be expected. Cosmetic surgical procedures such as the implantation of a high-polymer plastic prosthesis should be reserved for the most serious cases, particularly because of the element of doubt concerning compatibility and long-term results.

2. Mammary Hyperplasia

Pathogenesis. Mammary hyperplasia is a pubertal hypertrophy of one or both breasts (Fig. 87), ordinarily involving both the glandular and fatty tissue. The etiology is unclear, but may involve an exaggerated response to sex steroids; excessive prolactin stimulation has also been suggested. Extreme forms are marked by stretch pain and even necrosis; mastoptosis is common.

Diagnosis. External examination is generally sufficient. The usual hormone studies tend to be normal, with no appreciable elevation of estrogen or prolactin. If changes are unilateral, mammography is recommended to exclude organic disease.

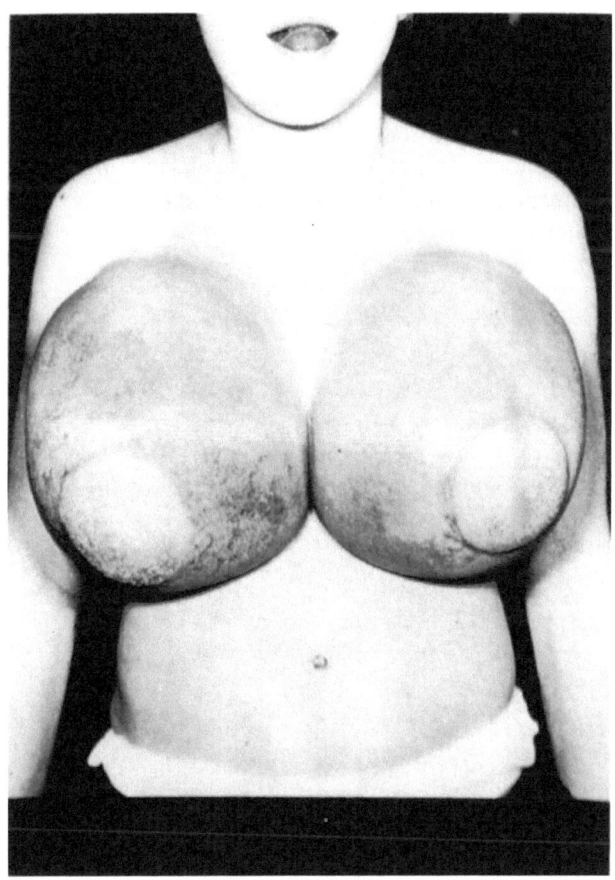

Fig. 87. Extreme hyperplasia of the breasts (14 years)

Treatment. Treatment, if necessary, is surgical and consists of reduction mammoplasty. Hormonal therapy is of little value.

3. Cystic Disease of the Breast

Pathogenesis. This is a quite common condition characterized by the appearance of one or many nodular cysts of the mammary parenchyma which result from proliferation or occlusion of the mammary ducts (Fig. 88). The cysts may vary from 1 or 2 mm to several centimeters in diameter and are tender to pressure. They are often filled with turbid fluid which is occasionally discharged from the nipple. The cysts may be confined to one sector, may involve one entire side, or both breasts. The disease is most common in the third and fourth decades of life; premenstrual swelling and painfulness are typical.

The cause is not entirely understood. As in cystic glandular hyperplasia of the endometrium, a chronic estrogen excess may play a role.

Diagnosis. Essentially the examination is restricted to local findings. It includes inspection and palpation, a check for nipple discharge, and examination of the regional lymph nodes, particularly the axillary nodes.

Mammography, galactoductography, and more recently, thermography can be useful aids, but excisional biopsy is often mandatory for establishing the diagnosis. Cystic disease must be differentiated from benign tumors of the breast such as fibroadenoma or lipoma, and particularly from mammary carcinoma. By itself, mammary pain may simply indicate mastodynia in the setting of premenstrual tension.

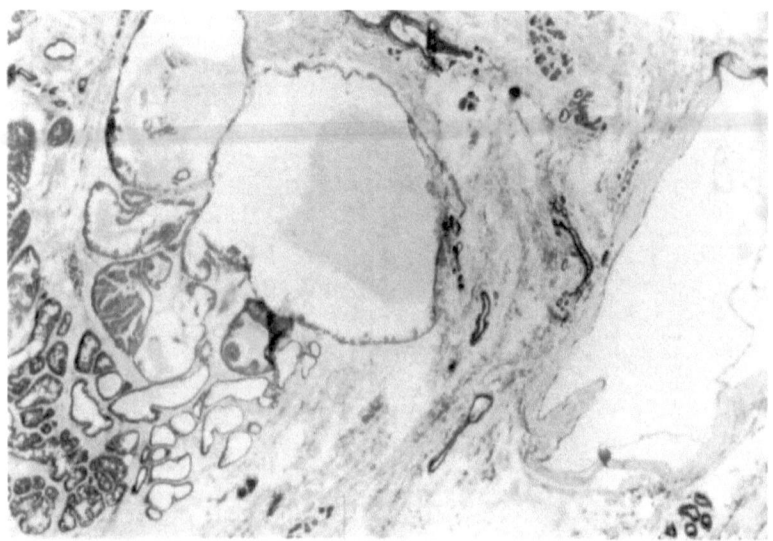

Fig. 88. Cystic disease of the breasts (Reclus' disease) (x 80)

Treatment. Excision is indicated in confirmed cases, perhaps combined with weakly virilizing androgens or, preferably, orally active gestagens such as Primolut N (Schering) in a dosage of 20 mg daily from cycle day 16 through 25. Other preparations such as Orgametril (Organon), Provera (Upjohn), and Danatrol (Winthrop) are also suitable. Recently, the percutaneous administration of progesterone (Progestagel, Besins-Iscovesca) has been recommended, but success with such treatment has been modest.

4. Galactorrhea

Pathogenesis. Galactorrhea refers to the unilateral or bilateral secretion of milk outside the lactation period (Fig. 89). This occurs physiologically during pregnancy and sometimes for a short time after weaning. In some cases bilateral galactorrhea is also observed during the use of oral contraceptives and psychotropic drugs, as well as in psychotic states, but its most likely cause is functional hyperprolactinemia or pituitary adenoma (see p 85). Unilateral galactorrhea may

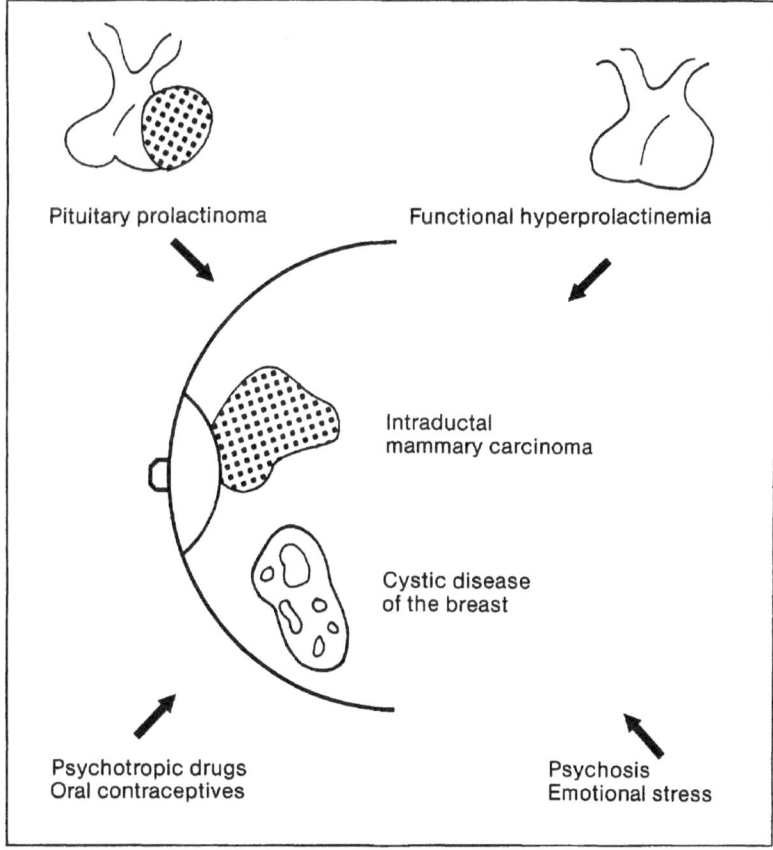

Fig. 89. Pathogenesis of galactorrhea

be associated with intraductal carcinoma; in such cases the secretion is often grayish in color, but may also be serous or bloody.

Diagnosis. On the one hand, the diagnosis must exclude local processes. This can be done by careful clinical examination and by mammography, galactoductography, or thermography; also, a smear should be prepared and examined histologically. On the other hand, it is necessary to perform multiple prolactin determinations in order to rule out an endocrine disturbance. If values are elevated, a roentgenographic or tomographic survey of the sella turcica is indicated so that a prolactinoma, if present, can be recognized as early as possible.

Treatment. Treatment is directed toward the cause; refer to the specific underlying disorder for suggestions. If organic causes can be excluded, galactorrhea is controlled most effectively with bromocriptin (Parlodel, Sandoz) in a dosage of 2.5–7.5 mg per day (see p 85).

References

ARCHER, D. F.: Current concepts of prolactin physiology in normal and abnormal conditions. Fertil. and Steril. **28**, 125 (1977).

APOSTOLAKIS, M., VOIGT, K. D.: Gonadotropine. Stuttgart: Thieme, 1965.

ARGONZ, J., DEL CASTILLO, E. B.: A syndrome characterized by estrogenic insufficiency, galactorrhea and decreased urinary gonadotropin. J. clin. Endocr. **13**, 79 (1953).

ARRATA, W. S. M., DE ALVAREZ, R. R.: The oversuppression syndrome. Amer. J. Obstet. Gynec. **112**, 1025 (1972).

BARRACLOUGH, C. A.: Central nervous regulation of the preovulatory release of FSH and LH from the pituitary gland. In: HAFEZ, E. S. E.: Human ovulation. Amsterdam: Elsevier, 1979.

BARR, M. L.: Das Geschlechtschromatin: In: OVERZIER, C.: Die Intersexualität. Stuttgart: Thieme, 1961.

BEHRMANN, S. J., KISTNER, R. W.: Progress in infertility, 2nd edn., New York: Little Brown, 1975.

BERGER, J.: Behandlung der Sterilität mit Cyclofenil. Schweiz. Z. Gynäk. Geburtsh. **3**, 209 (1972).

BESSER, G. M., MCNEILLY, A. S., ANDERSON, D. C., MARSHALL, J. C., HARSOULIS, P., HALL, R., ORMSTON, B. J., ALEXANDER, L., COLLINS, W. P.: Hormonal responses to synthetic luteinizing hormone and follicle-stimulating hormone-releasing hormone in man. Brit. Med. J. **3**, 267 (1972).

BESSER, G. M., EDWARDS, C. R. W.: Galactorrhea. Brit. med. J. **2**, 280 (1972).

BETTENDORF, G., INSLER, V.: Clinical application of human gonadotropins. Stuttgart: Thieme, 1970.

BICKENBACH, W., DÖRING, G. K.: Die Sterilität der Frau (4th edn.). Stuttgart: Thieme, 1969.

BIERICH, J. R.: Adrenogenitales Syndrom. In: OVERZIER, C.: Die Intersexualität. Stuttgart: Thieme, 1961.

BOHNET, H. G., DAHLEN, H. G., WUTTKE, W., SCHNEIDER, H. P. G.: Hyperprolactinemic anovulatory syndrome. J. clin. Endocr. Metab. **42**, 132 (1976).

BOSCHHANN, H. W.: Praktische Zytologie. Berlin: De Gruyter, 1960.

BREUER, H.: Steuerung, Biogenese und Stoffwechsel der Sexualhormone. Aesth. Med. **16**, 227 (1967).

BREUER, H., HAMEL, D., KRÜSKEMPER, H. L.: Methoden der Hormonbestimmung. Stuttgart: Thieme, 1975.

BROWN, J. B.: Oestrogens in the human female. In: CAREY, H. M.: Modern trends in human reproductive physiology, Vol. I, p. 49. London: Butterworth, 1963.

BROWN, J. B., MACLEOD, S. C., MACNAUGHTON, C., SMITH, M. A., SMITH, B.: A rapid method for measuring oestrogens in human urine using a semiautomatic extractor. J. Endocr. **42**, 5 (1968).

BUCHANAN, G. D., TREDWAY, D. R.: Hyperprolactinemia and ovulatory dysfunction. In: HAFEZ, E. S. E.: Human ovulation. Amsterdam: Elsevier, 1979.

CALI, R. W., PRATT, J. H.: Congenital absence of vagina. Amer. J. Obstet. Gynec. **100**, 752 (1968).

CARD, I.: The Chiari-Frommel syndrome: An experiment of nature. J. Obstet. Gynaec. Brit. Cwlth. **71**, 624 (1964).

CHALMERS, J. A.: Endometriosis. London: Butterworth, 1975.

COHEN, M. R., STEIN, J. F., KAYE, B. M.: Spinnbarkeit: A characteristic of cervical mucus. Fertil and Steril. **3**, 20 (1952).

CONDRAU, G.: Psychosomatik der Frauenheilkunde, 2nd edn., Bern: Huber, 1969

COOKE, I. D.: Clinics in Obstetrics and Gynaecology, Vol. 1: The management of infertility. London: Saunders, 1974.

CROSIGNANI, P. G., JAMES, V. H. T.: Recent Progress in Reproductive Endocrinology. New York: Academic Press, 1974.

CROSIGNANI, P. G., MISHELL, D. R.: Ovulation in the human. London: Academic Press, 1976.

CZYGAN, P. J.: Regulationsprinzipien der weiblichen Keimdrüsenfunktion. Fortschr. Geburtsh. Gynäk. Vol. 52, Basel: Karger, 1974.

DICZFALUSY, E., LAURITZEN, C.: Oestrogene beim Menschen. Berlin: Springer, 1961.

DODEK, O. I., KOTZ, H. L.: Syndrome of anovulation following the oral contraceptives. Amer. J. Obstet. Gynec. **98**, 1065 (1967).

CUNCAN, J. M.: Fecundity, fertility, sterility and allied topics. Edinburgh: Black, 1966.

ECKSTEIN, P.: Ovarian physiology in the nonpregnant female. In: ZUCKERMANN, S.: The ovary, Vol. I. New York: Academic Press, 1962.

FERIN, J., RENAER, M.: Treatment of anovulatory infertility with human menopausal gonadotropin followed by human chorionic gonadotropin. Amer. J. Obstet. Gynec. **101**, 439 (1968).

FIKENTSCHER, R., SEMM, K.: Die apparativ gesteuerte Eileiterdurchblasung. Geburtsh. Frauenheilk. **24**, 541 (1964).

FLUHMANN, C. F.: Dysmenorrhea. Clin. Obstet. Gynec. **6**, 718 (1963).

FORBES, A. P., HENNEMANN, P. H., GRISWALD, G. C., ALBRIGHT, F.: Syndrome characterized by galactorrhea, amenorrhea and low urinary FSH: Comparison with acromegaly and normal lactation. J. clin. Endocr. **14**, 265 (1965).

FRANGENHEIM, H.: Die Laparoskopie und Culdoskopie in der Gynäkologie. 2nd edn., Stuttgart: Thieme, 1971.

FRIEDRICH, F.: Klinik der Gelbkörperfunktion. Wien-München-Bern: W. Maudrich, 1975.

GAY, V. L.: The hypothalamus: Physiology and clinical use of releasing factors. Fertil. and Steril. **23**, 50 (1972).

GEMZELL, C. A., ROOS, P.: Pregnancies following treatment with human gonadotropins with special reference to the problem of multiple births. Amer. J. Obstet. Gynec. **94**, 490 (1966).

GOLD, J. J.: Gynecologic endocrinology, 2nd edn., New York: Harper & Row, 1975.

GOLDZIEHER, J. W.: Polycystic ovarian disease. In: Progress in infertility, S. J. Behrman and R. W. Kistner. Boston: Little, Brown, 1975.

GRANT, A.: Cervical hostility: Incidence, diagnosis and prognosis. Fertil. and Steril. **9**, 321 (1958).

GREENBLATT, R. B.: Ovulation (stimulation, suppression, detection). Philadelphia: Lippincott, 1966.

GREENBLATT, R. B.: Recent advances in endometriosis. Amsterdam: Excerpta Medica, 1976.

GREENBLATT, R. B., ROGERS, J., McDONOUGH, P. G., MAHESH, V. B.: The spectrum of gonadal dysgenesis. Amer. J. Obstet. Gynec. **98**, 151 (1967).

GREENBLATT, R. B., CONIFF, R. F.: Hirsutism and the Stein-Leventhal syndrome. Fertil. and Steril. **19**, 661 (1968).

GREENE, R., L. DALTON, K.: The premenstrual syndrome. Brit. med. J. 1007 (1953).

GROPP, A.: Untersuchung von Chromosomen. In: KÄSER, O., FRIEDBERG, V., OBER, K. G., THOMSEN, K., ZANDER, J.: Gynäkologie und Geburtshilfe, Vol. I. Stuttgart: Thieme, 1969.

GUAL, C., ROSEMBERG, E.: Hypothalamic hypophysiotropic hormones. Excerpta medica (Amst.) 1973.

HAFEZ, E. S. E.: Human ovulation. Amsterdam: Elsevier, 1979.

HAFEZ, E. S. E., REEL, J. R.: Hypothalamic hormones, New York: Wiley, 1974.

HAFEZ, E. S. E., THIBAULT, G. G.: The biology of spermatozoa. Basel: Karger, 1975.

HARRIS, G. W., DONOVAN, B. T.: The pituitary gland, Vol. I–III. London: Butterworth, 1966.

106

HELLINGA, G., LANGEDIJK, H. I. M.: Induction of menstruation, ovulation and pregnancy with Sexovid (F 6066). Acta endocr. Suppl. **119**, 222 (1967).

HUBINONT, P. O., L'HERMITE, M., ROBYN, C.: Clinical reproductive neuroendocrinology. Basel: Karger, 1977.

INGERSLEV, M.: Experience with Danazol in severe and extensive endometriosis. J. int. med. Res. **5**, Suppl. 3, 81 (1977).

INSLER, V., LUNENFELD, B.: Sterilität. Berlin: Grosse, 1977.

INSLER, V., MELMED, H., EICHENBRENNER, I., SERR, D. M., LUNENFELD, B.: The Cervical Score. Int. J. Gynec. Obstet. **10**, 223 (1972).

IRVINE, W. J.: Reproductive endocrinology. Edinburgh: Livingstone, 1970.

ISRAEL, S. L.: Premenstrual tension. In: ISRAEL, S. L.: Menstrual disorders and sterility. New York: Harper & Row, 1967.

JAFFE, B. M., BEHRMANN, H. R.: Methods of radioimmunoassay. New York: Academic Press, 1974.

JAMES, V. H. T., SERIO, M., GIUSTI, G., MARTINI, L.: The endocrine function of the human adrenal cortex. London: Academic Press, 1978.

JONES, G. S.: The luteal phase defect. Fertil. and Steril. **27**, 351 (1976).

JUNKMANN, K.: Die Androgenbildung im Ovar. In: NOWAKOWSKI, H.: Moderne Entwicklungen auf dem Gestagengebiet. Berlin: Springer, 1960.

KAISER, R.: Hormonale Behandlung von Zyklusstörungen (5th edn.). Stuttgart: Thieme, 1975.

KASTIN, A. J., SCHALLY, A. V., GUAL, C., ARIMURA, A.: Release of LH and FSH after administration of synthetic LH-releasing hormone. J. clin. Endocr. **34**, 753 (1972).

KELLER, P. J.: Hypophysäre Gonadotropine. Basel: Karger, 1971.

KELLER, P. J.: Physiologie des menstruellen Zyklus. Gynäk. Rdsch. **3**, 13 (1973).

KELLER, P. J.: Amenorrhoe, Schweiz. med. Wschr. **106**, 1154 (1976).

KELLER, P. J.: A pituitary function test with synthetic LH-releasing hormone J. Obstet. Gynaec. Brit. Cwlth. **80**, 71 (1973).

KELLER, P. J.: Ovulationsauslösung durch Sexualsteroide. In: KÄSER, O., OBOLENSKY, W.: Ovulation und Ovulationsauslösung, Bern: Huber, 1975.

KELLER, P. J.: Ovar. In: LABHART, A.: Klinik der inneren Sekretion, 3rd, edn., Berlin, Heidelberg, New York: Springer, 1978.

KELLER, P. J.: Female Infertility. Contr. Gynec. Obstet., Vol. 4. Basel: Karger, 1978.

KEPP, R., STÄMMLER, H. J.: Lehrbuch der Gynäkologie (11. Ed.). Stuttgart: Thieme, 1974.

KERN-BONTKE, E.: Kerngeschlechtsdiagnostik. In: KÄSER, O., FRIEDBERG, V., OBER, K. G., THOMSEN, K., ZANDER, J.: Gynäkologie und Geburtshilfe, Bd. I; S. 884. Stuttgart: Thieme, 1969.

KISTNER, R. W.: Management of endometriosis in the infertile patient. Fertil. and Steril **26**, 1151 (1975).

KISTNER, R. W., PATTON, G. W.: Atlas of infertility surgery. New York: Little Brown, 1975.

KLEINBERG, D. L., NOEL, G. L., FRANTZ, A. G.: Galactorrhea: A study of 235 cases including 48 with pituitary tumors. New Engl. J. Med. **296**, 589 (1977).

KLOPPER, A., MICHIE, E. A., BROWN, J. B.: A method for determination of urinary pregnanediol. J. Endocr. **12**, 209 (1955).

KÜCHMEISTER, H., BARTELHEIMER, H., JORES, A.: Klinische Funktionsdiagnostik (3rd edn.). Stuttgart: Thieme, 1967.

LABHART, A.: Klinik der inneren Sekretion. 3rd edn. Berlin, Heidelberg, New York: Springer, 1978.

LAURITZEN, C., VAN KEEP, P. A.: Estrogens therapy. The benefits and risks. Basel: Karger, 1978.

LEHMANN, W. D., LAURITZEN, Ch.: Kombinierter Funktionstest mit Dexamethason und Choriongonadotropin zur Diagnose androgenbildender Ovarialtumoren. Geburtsh. u. Frauenheilk. **32**, 913 (1972).

LEVENTHAL, M. L., The Stein-Leventhal syndrome. Amer. J. Obstet. Gynec. **76**, 825 (1958).

LLOYD, S. J., JOSIMOVICH, J. B., ARCHER, D. F.: Amenorrhea and galactorrhea: Results of therapy with 2-brom-ergocryptine (CB 154). Amer. J. Obstet. Gynec. **122**, 85 (1975).

LUDWIG, H., TAUBER, P. F.: Human fertilization. Stuttgart: Thieme, 1978.

LUKAS, K. H.: Die Dysmenorrhoe. Geburtsh. Gynäk. **163**, 1 (1965).

LUNENFELD, B.: Treatment of anovulation by human gonadotropins. J. int. Fed. Gynaec. Obstet. **1**, 153 (1963).

LUNENFELD, B., GLEZERMAN, M.: Auswahl und Abklärung der Patientinnen zur Ovulationsauslösung. Bern: Huber, 1975.

LYNDA, L. E.: Gynaecologic endocrinology of adolescence. Clin. Obstet. Gynaec. **9**, 759 (1966).

MASTROIANNI, L.: Ovulation. Clin. Obstet. Gynaec. **10**, 345 (1967).

MEYER, J. E., FELDMANN, H.: Anorexia nervosa. Stuttgart: Thieme, 1965.

MORICARD, R., FERIN, J.: L'ovulation. Paris: Masson, 1969.

MORRIS, J.: The syndrome of testicular feminization in male pseudohermaphroditism. Amer. J. Obstet. Gynec. **65**, 1192 (1953).

MOTTA, M., CROSIGNANI, P. G., MARTINI, L.: Hypothalamic hor hormones. New York: Academic Press, 1975.

MÜLLER, J.: Untersuchungsmethoden der Nebennierenrinden-Funktion. In: LABHART, A.: Klinik der inneren Sekretion. Berlin: Springer, 1978.

NADER, S., MASHITER, K., DOYLE, F. M., JOPLIN, G. F.: Galactorrhea, hyperprolactinemia and pituitary tumors in the female. Clin. Endocr. **5**, 245 (1975).

NAEF, J. C. De: Clinical endocrine cytology. New York: Hoeber, 1967.

NEWTON, J., COLLINS, W., KILPATRICK, M., PYKE, J.: Studies on synthetic LH releasing hormone. J. Reprod. Fertil. **35**, 622 (1973).

NOCKE, W., LEYENDECKER, G.: Neue Erkenntnisse über die endokrine Regulation der Ovarialfunktion. Gynäk. Rdsch. **12**, 58 (1972).

NOWAKOWSKI, H.: Erkrankungen der Nebennieren. In: JORES, A., NOWAKOWSKI, H.: Praktische Endokrinologie 3rd edn. Stuttgart: Thieme, 1968.

OTTO, H., MINNECKER, C., SPAETHE, R.: Synacthen-Kurztest zur Beurteilung der Nebennierenrindenfunktion. Dtsch. med. Wschr. **91**, 943 (1966).

OVERZIER, C.: Die Intersexualität. In: KÄSER, O., FRIEDBERG, V., OBER, K. G., THOMSEN, K., ZANDER, J.: Gynäkologie und Geburtshilfe, Vol. I, Stuttgart: Thieme, 1969.

PAULSEN, C. A.: Estrogen assays in clinical medicine. Seattle: Univ. Washington Press, 1965.

PHILIP, J., SELE, V., TROLLE, D.: Primary amenorrhea: A study of 101 cases. Fertil. and Steril. **16**, 795 (1965).

PLOTZ, J.: Der Wert der Basaltemperatur für die Diagnose der Menstruationsstörungen. Arch. Gynäk. **177**, 521 (1950).

POLISHUK, W. Z., PALTI, Z., RABAU, E., LUNENFELD, B., DAVID, A.: Pregnancy in a case of Sheehan's syndrome following treatment with human gonadotropins. J. Obstet. Gynaec. Brit. Cwlth. **72**, 778 (1965).

POZO, E. DEL, BRUN DEL RE, R., VARGA, L., FRIESEN, H.: The inhibition of prolactin secretion in man by CB-154 (2-Br-alpha-ergocryptine). J. clin. Endocr. **35**, 768 (1972).

PRADER, A.: Störungen der Geschlechtsdifferenzierung (Intersexualität). In: LABHART, A.: Klinik der inneren Sekretion (3rd edn.). Berlin: Springer, 1978.

PRADER, A.: Wachstum und Entwicklung. In: LABHART, A.: Klinik der inneren Sekretion (3rd edn.). Berlin: Springer, 1978.

PRILL, H. J.: Klimax praecox, klimax tarda (ein statistischer Vergleich). Geburtsh. u. Frauenheilk. **26**, 883 (1966).

RAKOFF, A. E.: Psychogenic factors in anovulatory women. Hormonal patterns in women with ovarian dysfunction of psychogenic origin. Fertil. and Steril. **13**, (1962).

RAJ, S. G., THOMPSON, I. E., BERGER, M. J., TAYMOR, M. L.: Clinical aspects of the polycystic ovary syndrome. Obstet. Gynec. **49**, 552 (1977).

ROSEMBERG, E., NWE, T. T.: Induction of ovulation with human postmenopausal gonadotropin. Fertil. and Steril. **19**, 197 (1968).

ROSEMBERG, E.: Gonadotropin therapy in female infertility. Excerpta medica (Amst.) 1973.

108

Ross, P.: Human follicle stimulating hormone. Acta endocrinol [Suppl.] (Kbh.) 131 (1968).

Rodbard, D.: Mechanics of ovulation. J. clin. Endocr. **28**, 849 (1968).

Ryan, K. J.: Steroid metabolism in the human ovary. In: Marcus, St. L., Marcus, C. C.: Adv. Obstet. Gynec., Vol. I. Baltimore: Williams & Wilkins, 1967.

Rybo, G.: Clinical and experimental studies on menstrual blood loss. Acta obstet. gynaec. scand. **45**, 7 (1966).

Sato, T., Ibuki, Y., Hirono, M., Igarashi, M., Matsumoto, S.: Induction of ovulation with Sexovid (Compound F 6066) and its mode of action. Fertil. and Steril. **20**, 965 (1969).

Saxena, B. B., Beling, C. G., Gandy, H. M.: Gonadotropins. New York: Wiley, 1972.

Schally, A. V., Kastin, A. J., Arimura, A.: Hypothalamic follicle-stimulating hormone (FSH) and luteinizing hormone (LH)-regulating hormone: Structure, physiology and clinical studies. Fertil. and Steril. **22**, 703 (1971).

Schally, A. V., Kastin, A. J., Arimura, A.: The hypothalamus and reproduction. Am. J. Obstet. Gynec. **114**, 423 (1972).

Schellen, T.: Releasing factors and gonadotropic hormones in male & female sterility. Radioimmunoassays as diagnostic tools in gynecology & andrology. Ghent: Medikon, 1975.

Schindler, A. E.: Bromoergocryptine for ovulation induction. In: Hafez, E. S. E.: Human ovulation. Amsterdam: Elsevier, 1979.

Schmidt-Elmendorff, H.: Klinische und experimentelle Ergebnisse mit dem Ovulationsauslöser Fertodur (Cyclofenil). Geburtsh. u. Frauenheilk. **31**, 693 (1971).

Schmidt-Elmendorff, H., Kaemmerling, R.: Vergleichende klinische Untersuchung von Clomiphen, Cyclofenil und Epimestrol. Geburtsh. u. Frauenheilk. **37**, 531 (1977).

Schwenk, A.: Die Vorbereitung der Fortpflanzungsfunktion von der Kindheit bis zur Pubertät und ihre Störungen. In: Käser, O., Friedberg, V., Ober, K. G., Thomsen, K., Zander, J.: Gynäkologie und Geburtshilfe, Vol. I. Stuttgart: Thieme, 1969.

Semm, K.: Pelviskopie und Hysteroskopie. Stuttgart: Schattauer, 1976.

Sherman, B. M., Korenmann, S. G.: Hormonal characteristics of the human menstrual cycle throughout reproductive life. J. clin. Invest. **55**, 699 (1975).

Siegler, S., Siegler, A. M.: Evaluation of the basal body temperature. An analysis of 1012 basal body temperature recordings. Fertil. and Steril. **2**, 287 (1951).

Southam, A. L.: Disorders of menstruation. Clin. Obstet. Gynaec. **9**, 779 (1966).

Stämmler, H. J.: Gynäkologische Hormontherapie in der Praxis. Planegg: Selecta, 1976.

Stämmler, H. J.: Fibel der gynäkologischen Endokrinologie (2nd edn.). Stuttgart: Thieme, 1969.

Stein, J. F.: Wedge resection of the ovaries: The Stein-Leventhal-syndrome. In: Greenblatt, R. B.: Ovulation. Philadelphia: Lippincott, 1966.

Tamm, J.: Testosteron. Stuttgart: Thieme, 1968.

Tanner, J. M.: Puberty. In: McLaren, A.: Advances in reproductive physiology. New York: Logos Press, London: Academic Press, 1967.

Tausk, M.: Pharmakologie der Hormone. Stuttgart: Thieme, 1970.

Ufer, J.: Hormontherapie in der Frauenheilkunde. 5th edn. Berlin: De Gruyter, 1978.

Van Keep, P. A., Lauritzen, C.: Estrogens in the post-menopause. Basel: Karger, 1975.

Van Keep, P. A., Lauritzen, C.: Ageing and estrogens. Basel: Karger, 1973.

Varga, L., Wenner, R., Pozo, E. Del: Treatment of galactorrhea-amenorrhea syndrome with Br-ergocryptine (CB-154): Restoration of ovulatory function and fertility. Amer. J. Obstet. Gynec. **117**, 75 (1973).

Vasterling, H. W.: Praktische Spermatologie. Stuttgart: Thieme, 1960.

Wld. Hlth. Org. Colloquium Geneva 1972: Cervical mucus in human reproduction. Copenhagen: Scriptor, 1973.

Young, M. D., Blackmore, W. P.: The use of Danazol in the management of endometriosis. J. int. med. Res. 5, Suppl. 3, 86 (1977).

Zander, J.: Der menstruelle Zyklus. In: Käser, O., Friedberg, V., Ober, K. G., Thomsen, K., Zander, J.: Gynäkologie und Geburtshilfe, Vol. I. Stuttgart: Thieme, 1969.

ZANDER, J., HOLZMANN, K.: Störungen des menstruellen Zyklus und ihre Behandlung. In: KÄSER, O., FRIEDBERG, V., OBER, K. G., THOMSEN, K., ZANDER, J.: Gynäkologie und Geburtshilfe, Vol. I, p. 315. Stuttgart: Thieme, 1969.

ZUSPAN, K. J., ZUSPAN, F. P.: Basal body temperature. In: HAFEZ, E. S. E.: Human ovulation. Amsterdam: Elsevier, 1979.

Subject Index

Functional Morphologic Changes in Female Sex Organs Induced by Exogenous Hormones

Editor: G. Dallenbach-Hellweg

1980. 139 figures, 42 tables. XV, 234 pages
ISBN-13: 978-3-540-10341-7

With contributions by numerous experts

The significance of the interplay between morphology and function is nowhere more evident than in the field of gynecopathology. The wide use of exogenous hormones, particularly as contraceptive agents in healthy young women, necessitates a clear understanding of their mode of action and the structural changes they cause.

This volume contains studies on the functional and morphological changes in female sex organs following administration of estrogen, of gestagen, and of a combination of hormones. The studies were conducted by researchers the world over, allowing observations and results from many different regions to be compared and discussed. They will aid in the recognition of adverse reactions and in the development of methods to prevent them.

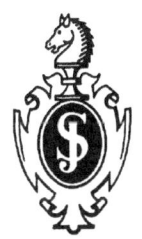
Springer-Verlag
Berlin
Heidelberg
New York

Carbohydrate Metabolism in Pregnancy and the Newborn 1978

Editors: H. W. Sutherland, J. M. Stowers
1979. 95 figures, 177 tables. XIV, 558 pages
ISBN-13: 978-3-540-10341-7

Clinical Management of Mother and Newborn

Editor: G. F. Marx
1979. 30 figures, 44 tables. XIV, 274 pages
ISBN-13: 978-3-540-10341-7

D. Fanta

Hormone Therapy of Acne

Clinical and Experimental Principles
Revised translation of "Akne. Klinische und experimentelle
Grundlagen zur Hormontherapie."
1980. 25 figures, 21 tables. VIII, 91 pages
Wien – New York: Springer-Verlag
ISBN-13: 978-3-540-10341-7

B. J. Masterson

Manual of Gynecologic Surgery

With contributions by K. E. Krantz, W. J. Cameron, J. W. Daly,
J. A. Fayez, E. W. Franklin
Illustrator: D. McKeown
1979. 204 figures, 192 in color, 12 tables. XV, 256 pages
(Comprehensive Manuals of Surgical Specialties)
ISBN-13: 978-3-540-10341-7

Perinatal Pathology

With contributions by M. Bibbo, C. Bron, W.-W. Höpker,
J. P. Kraehenbuhl, B. Ohlendorf, L. Olding, S. Panem,
B. Sandstedt, H. Soma, B. Sordat
Editors: E. Grundmann, W. H. Kirsten
1979. 88 figures, 34 tables. VI, 218 pages
(Current Topics in Pathology, Vol. 66)
ISBN-13: 978-3-540-10341-7

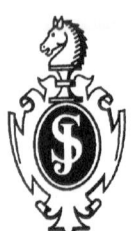

Springer-Verlag
Berlin
Heidelberg
New York

Placental Proteins

Editors: A. Klopper, T. Chard
1979. 65 figures, 36 tables. X, 171 pages
ISBN-13: 978-3-540-10341-7